C000084509

Behaviour
and Rehabilitation

Behaviour and Rehabilitation

behavioural treatment for long-stay patients

by
Richard J Butler BSc MSc ABPsS
Principal Clinical Psychologist
High Royds Hospital Menston W. Yorkshire
and
Gerald Rosenthall RMN SRN
Charge Nurse
Stanley Royd Hospital Wakefield, W. Yorkshire

Second Edition

WRIGHT
Bristol
1985

Published by
John Wright & Sons Ltd, Techno House, Redcliffe Way, Bristol BS1 6NX, England

First edition, 1978
Second edition, 1985

British Library Cataloguing in Publication Data
Butler, Richard J. L.
 Behaviour and rehabilitation: behavioural
 treatment for long-stay patients.—2nd ed.
 1. Behaviour therapy 2. Psychiatric hospital
 care—Great Britain 3. Psychiatric nursing
 —Great Britain
 I. Title II. Rosenthal, Gerald
 616.89′16 RC489.B4

ISBN 0 7236 0824 5

Typeset by
Severntype Repro Services Ltd,
Market Street, Wotton-under-Edge, Glos.

Printed in Great Britain by
John Wright & Sons (Printing) Ltd
at The Stonebridge Press,
Bristol BS4 5NU

Preface

Traditional psychiatric hospitals contain an enormous number of long-stay patients; people who have spent at least two but usually many more years in the confines of the hospital environment and who show a range of behaviour problems varying in severity. For such patients the past has been a long and monotonous routine, interspersed with unsuccessful attempts at treatment, and the future has, until recently, looked fairly bleak.

Patients are thus construed as 'failures', and their often bizarre behaviour perplexes those who care for them. However, why patients behave as they do may not be quite the mystery some would have us believe. Adopting a 'behavioural model' which is derived from general learning principles, offers us a way of understanding a patient's present behavioural repertoire. Applying behavioural procedures enables change to occur: patients learn to develop or build more appropriate behaviour into their repertoire and reduce their inappropriate behaviour.

Such procedures have been given a number of terms: 'behaviour modification', 'behavioural psychotherapy' and 'behavioural treatment'. These terms are interchangeable and will be used as such throughout this book.

Over the last 15 years or so behaviour modification has become increasingly more popular in the treatment of long-stay patients. Applied initially in American institutions, it was found such treatment could greatly improve the lot of long-stay patients and in some cases it enabled them eventually to leave the hospital and live in the community again.

Behavioural treatment, to be effective, relies heavily on structuring the relationships between therapist and patient. As nurses are in more contact with patients than any other professional body, they become key figures in the patients' treatment. During our work at Stanley Royd Hospital, Wakefield, we became aware of the lack of a suitable British textbook for nurses who were interested in developing their therapeutic skills through behavioural treatment. Together with our experience in encouraging nurses to explore their potential as therapists, we were motivated to write this book. Since it was published in 1978, many changes have taken place in the Mental Health Services of the United

v

Kingdom. Amongst these changes have been the implementation of the Mental Health Act (1983), the reduction in numbers of staff and patients in large psychiatric hospitals, a growing number of nurses working in the community outside the hospital and the gradual transfer of patients from hospitals to accommodation in the community.

Many factors have effected these environmental changes. In behavioural terms we would describe them as the 'antecedents' which influence 'behaviour'. Amongst these antecedents have been the humanitarian desire to provide a more natural setting in which long-stay psychiatric patients can live, and the economic aspects of the environment which have stimulated these changes and govern the rate of their implementation. (We all live in a 'Token Economy' world!)

The introduction of the 'Nursing Process' is particularly welcome, for the concept of behavioural treatment can only be successfully practised in the context of 'assessment' of the patient's problems; designing a 'programme' to reduce or eradicate those problems; 'implementing' the treatment programme; and 'evaluating' the results of the treatment programme.

However, despite the many favourable changes which have taken place, some aspects of psychiatry have not radically altered. The nature and quality of the psychiatric patient's problems remain unchanged. There has not been any major alteration in the physical treatments available to these people and the provision of residential accommodation in the community outside the boundary walls of a hospital will not ensure that they will be protected from the conditions which produce 'institutionalization'.

Adequate training in preparing patients for discharge from hospital is still necessary. The growing use of behavioural treatment has proved to be the most effective means of providing that preparation. Because the process of rehabilitation is a continuous one, liaison with social workers and carers in the community at an early stage, well before a patient's discharge, is essential. Their introduction and continuing social contact with the patient, as well as their understanding of the approaches to the patient in the existing training programme, will help to ensure a smooth transition from hospital to the community. Once outside the hospital and living in less confining circumstances, the need for a regular daily routine is important if deterioration of that person's condition is to be avoided. When that daily routine has been established, the quality of his life needs to be developed and maintained.

Sadly, we know in our hearts that many patients in hospital will never be able to leave it. The severity of their problems excludes the possibility of them living any realistic form of independent life in the community. Amongst that growing population are the elderly people, now termed the 'Elderly Severely Mentally Infirm'. The target of their form of rehabilitation is to maintain their appropriate behaviours already in existence, to organize a suitable environment which will help to preserve their physical, mental and social assets for as long as possible, and to remember that whether the therapist is a nurse, a doctor, a social worker or any other carer involved in the treatment of an individual person, the most important instrument of therapy is the therapist.

R.J.B.
G.R.

Acknowledgements

For a number of years we worked as members of a research team involved in various aspects of behavioural treatment with long-stay psychiatric patients. This book owes much to what we learned over those years and to our attempts at training nurses interested in such work. We are indebted to all those who were involved in the preparation of this manuscript.

We wish to express special thanks to Professor Gwynne Jones, Dr John Hall and Dr Roger Baker for their advice; to Jan Needham, Rosemary Kneebone and Jackie Stainer for typing the various drafts; to Peter Andrews, the Nursing Officer of the Rehabilitation Unit; to all the nursing staff involved in the programme for their willingness to try out new techniques; and to all the patients, without whom none of this would have been possible. The procedures described are based largely on the research of scores of workers in the USA and Britain and we owe much to their vigorous and inventive efforts. They are cited throughout the text and we are indebted to them all.

Contents

SECTION I
THE LONG-STAY PATIENT

Chapter 1

THE PATIENT'S CONDITION

The sight of a group of patients dishevelled in appearance, lacking in interaction and largely inactive is one all too common on the long-stay wards, and the corridors, of a psychiatric hospital. These individuals are resident in hospital as a result of three interacting variables:
1. The patient's condition, or illness, for which he was originally admitted and from which he may still be largely suffering. For most, especially those hospitalized for over 10 years, the diagnosis is one of *schizophrenia,* a devastating and incapacitating illness.
2. The effect of living in hospital for many years. Patients showing little or no improvement in their condition over the first two years of hospitalization are often termed 'chronic' and transferred to a long-stay ward. Adapting to living a life in hospital creates a wealth of new, often inappropriate, behaviour.
3. The failure to respond to various treatment methods heralded at or around the time of their admission. As treatment techniques 20–30 years ago were far less sophisticated than those of today, the incidence of non-response was higher than at present. However, even today there are patients finding their way onto the long-stay wards.

Section 1 deals with these three variables, emphasizing how each may result in characteristic behaviours. A patient's behaviour must inevitably be the result of an interaction of all three variables. That they are given a chapter each serves only as a way of exploring the wide range of behaviours exhibited by long-stay patients.

We concentrate on behaviour rather than diagnosis. Behaviour is observable, whereas diagnosis is a subjective judgement. A diagnosis

1

can be remarkably unreliable. For example, schizophrenia is diagnosed much more frequently in the USA than in Britain, partly because American psychiatrists appear far more ready to detect abnormality, and also because of an American attitude that even a 'trace' of schizophrenia is sufficient to label a person schizophrenic. Neither is the diagnosis consistent among different psychiatrists in the same country. This is hardly surprising, for diagnosis relies on the subjective assessment of a whole range of individual behaviours and the recognition that they reflect a familiar pattern of abnormality and the labelling of the pattern as fitting into a particular category. Assigning labels to patients may blind us to the patient's special difficulties. We must therefore begin to look at the behaviours our patients display. Behaviours are readily observable, they can be objectively assessed and, as will be demonstrated, are potentially amenable to modification.

In order to describe the behaviour of long-stay patients, we begin by looking at behaviours resulting from disturbance in psychological functioning. We can view disturbance as arising in five functions:
1. Perception
2. Thought and speech
3. Will
4. Emotion
5. Motor behaviour

1. PERCEPTION

The number of stimuli impinging on our sense organs at any one time is enormous. We manage usually not to be overwhelmed by incoming stimulation from the eyes, ears, nose, taste buds and tactile receptors because we develop means of selecting out what seems important. We develop the ability to attend to particular aspects of the events going on around us, whilst 'filtering out' other events or stimuli. Each of us discovers ways of imposing our own structure on the environment. A child does not begin to understand what a table is, for example, until he can impose his own discriminations on the object. He may construe it as *solid* rather than *liquid, hard* rather than *soft* and so on. Only when he can begin to discriminate the table as something, rather than something else, does the object become meaningful to the child. Such discriminations are also *predictive.* So when we construe a table as solid rather than liquid we are essentially predicting that if something is placed upon it, it will stay on the surface and not be submerged. If we construe it as hard rather than soft we predict stubbing our toe into it will cause our toe to be crushed rather than the table give in. Thus the table becomes meaningful to us through applying our discriminations. In this way we learn to understand our environment, not just the physical environment but the psychological environment too. So when we construe someone as honest rather than dishonest we are predicting that if we lend him money we shall get it back. Each of us sees what confronts us, our environments, ourselves in a unique way. We have a unique system of discriminations we impose on the environment. We differ from others in how we perceive and interpret a situation, what we consider important about it, what we consider its implications and so forth.

When we are unable to form discriminations or construe an event, that event is meaningless to us. For example, a non-mechanic might have only a very limited number of discriminations available to him to help understand what lies under the bonnet of his car. He may be able to construe the engine as dirty rather than clean and not working rather than working but without more elaborate constructions, the engine is in the main not understood by him.

Sometimes, it seems, long-stay patients have difficulty in construing or imposing meaning on their environment. This is particularly so in their understanding of other people. It is as if they are overwhelmed by stimulation, unable to select or discriminate anything meaningful from what confronts them.

This may have a number of effects on the patient's behaviour:

(a) *Distractability.* A patient may have difficulty in concentrating on one thing for any length of time. One patient described this when he said, 'I can't concentrate. It's diversion of attention that troubles me—the sounds are coming through to me but I feel my mind cannot cope with everything. It is difficult to concentrate on any one sound . . . it's like trying to do two or three different things at one time.'

(b) *Withdrawal.* Other people, or the psychological environment, is often the area which lacks meaning for the patient. He is unable to construe others adequately and therefore is unable to predict or anticipate their behaviour and reactions. Avoiding others is therefore an option patients take so as to reduce being confronted by situations they find difficult to understand. This a patient may do in various ways such as sitting alone in a corner, avoiding looking or communicating with others, becoming inactive during ward activities and turning away, shutting his eyes or failing to respond when asked a question.

(c) *Hallucinations.* These are experiences perceived by the patient in the absence of any sensory stimulation. It is as if the patient construes internal stimuli as though they had an external origin. Hallucinations are quite different from *illusions* which are misinterpretations of external stimuli. On a dark evening, for example, we may wrongly interpret a shadow as an animal or strange figure. We are 'fooled' into believing something, which in reality, is something quite different.

Hallucinations take many forms and can occur in any of the senses:

(i) *Auditory hallucinations,* where patients complain of hearing noises, are by far the most common type. They range from buzzing or whistling noises to screaming, laughing and distinct voices. They also vary in quality; some being clear, others so vague the patient has difficulty in describing them, some voices being familiar to the patient, others strange. They are often hostile and abusive, sometimes neutral but rarely reassuring. The voices may talk about the patient or instruct him to do various things, and some patients even report hearing their own thoughts being spoken aloud.

(ii) *Visual hallucinations* are relatively uncommon in long-stay patients but when they do occur they are not alone—there is usually disturbance in one or other of the senses as well. They vary from 'seeing' flashes of light to organized perceptions of people and animals. Thus a patient may complain, for example, of seeing faces on the wall when in fact the wall is blank and free from pictures.

(iii) *Hallucinations of smell and taste* usually become apparent when a patient starts to complain about odd tastes or smells when none are present. Some of the most frequent are complaints of rotting odours, of gas being pumped into the room, of food tasting bad or of being poisoned with arsenic.

(iv) *Bodily or tactile hallucinations* may occur, in which the individual complains of being touched or assaulted. Patients may, for example, complain that their flesh is being torn away, that a machine has been inserted in their body, that a tapeworm is eating the brain away or that the mind feels 'like it has been rubbed raw with sandpaper'.

The effects these hallucinations may have on a patient's behaviour are quite varied:

(α) He may become so preoccupied with the hallucinations that he withdraws from the environment and consequently fails to interact with other people. When asked a question, he may come out of the preoccupied state but is unable to answer the question, often being unaware of what has been asked him.

(β) There may be odd behaviour as a result of reacting to the hallucination. Impulsive behaviour such as breaking a window or hitting another person may result as the patient obeys what his 'voices' tell him to do. He may laugh out loud or answer back the voices, so that to an observer he may be seen as 'talking to himself'.

(γ) Hallucinations may continually interfere with thinking so the person's speech disintegrates and becomes incomprehensible.

(δ) A patient may try to explain the origin of the sensations by attributing them to machines, spirits, X-rays or some other part of the body.

2. THOUGHT AND SPEECH

We perceive a person's thoughts, ideas and beliefs by what he says and to a lesser extent by what he writes. Thus when thinking processes become disturbed, as they do in schizophrenia, they must be interpreted from the individual's speech or his writing.

A most characteristic feature of long-stay patients is the lack of speech. There is relatively little patient–patient or staff–patient interaction when compared to other groups of people. Most of the speech uttered by patients is not self initiated—that is, it usually occurs as a response to a question, direction or comment from another person, most frequently a nurse.

When patients do speak, and there are the exceptional patients who talk quite freely and spontaneously, they often reveal disturbances in the production of speech, the content of thought and the form of speech.

Production of speech

Where speech is completely absent, the patient is said to be mute. He may grunt and possibly laugh, communicate by gesture or writing, but fails to utter a comprehensible word. Some may be evasive and turn away when questioned. *Monosyllabic speech* may be shown by patients who are not completely mute. They answer questions with a 'Yes', 'No', or 'Don't know' but rarely add anything else. *Stunted speech* is said to occur when patients are incapable of stringing many words or sentences together and speech then becomes short and terse. For example, a patient might answer 'like pictures' to the question 'What did you think of those pictures?'

One must be careful in attributing 'abnormality' where a patient's speech is stunted or monosyllabic. The content of a conversation with a patient is often dependent on the nurse for it is she who initiates and hence decides upon what to talk about. Thus the patient may answer in monosyllables because of a lack of interest in the topic being discussed. Where there is a lack of speech production it is difficult to know whether the thought process is abnormal, or whether thinking processes themselves are normal but the expression disturbed. The speech of long-term patients may also vary from normality in volume (either very quiet or rarely loud utterances), in rhythm (often extremely slow) and in associated affect (usually a monotonous and expressionless speech with a failure to emphasize key words).

Content of thought

When the contents of a patient's thinking become bizarre he is said to be deluded. More formally, a *delusion* is 'a false unshakable belief which is out of keeping with the patient's cultural and educational background'. A delusion is more than just a false belief, it is an absolute and inconvertible conviction about the truth of a proposition. The deluded person believes with an unshakable conviction that, for example, he is being interfered with by X-ray machines. He is consequently not amenable to reason or persuasion about the falseness of his conviction. The belief must also be seen to be out of keeping with the beliefs of his own culture. Two further characteristics of delusions are that they often preoccupy the patient's thinking and that they are usually absurd and impossible. The commonest delusional themes are of persecution, grandiosity and interference. With the former the person may believe he is being persecuted by someone such as a member of his family or a group of people such as the police or the Jews. He may feel he is being watched or followed and every move or gesture a person in the near vicinity makes may be interpreted by him to mean he is being plotted against. He may feel people are taking nerves out of his body, poisoning his food, trying to kill him or robbing him of his just inheritance.

Grandiose delusions are where the patient believes he is some great person, such as the King of England or the Virgin Mary; or is endowed with great skill or power, such as a well-known painter or inventor. The extent of the grandiosity varies: one patient, for example, believed that he was the Lord, born in the year 1, whilst another believed he owned a garage full of cars.

Delusions of interference are where an individual believes that his person is being tampered with. For example, a patient might complain of someone taking his blood away when he's asleep, of making his face ugly, or that he is being controlled by cosmic rays.

Form of speech

The speech of a normal person has some degree of logical association or continuity between successive phrases and sentences, and ideas are expressed with a view to obtaining some goal. Long-stay patients often show disturbances of association or of relevance, which can take several forms.

(*a*) *Thought blocking.* This describes the sudden arrest of a train of thought, as if the mind had just gone blank. If speaking, the patient is left speechless and after a period of time he often resumes with an entirely new thought. Thought blocking can also interfere with actions, so that a patient may take longer to react to a question than would normally be expected.

(*b*) *Unusual associations.* The normal process whereby thoughts and ideas are strung together becomes disturbed, and so an association between one idea and the next is not obvious. One patient described this process thus: 'I started a train of ideas which finished itself off or got lost in a tangle of cross associations . . . I could not direct its course at all'.

It seems as though thoughts spark off other thoughts which have only a tenuous logical link with each other. The following dialogues illustrate this:

(i)   Patient   'I thought it was wrong but I can't do much wrong.'
        Nurse   'Why can't you do anything wrong?'
        Patient   'I'm a law unto myself . . . the white coat.'
(ii)   Patient   'She's not big enough.'
        Nurse   'What do you mean?'
        Patient   'That piece of cake I had last night.'

This type of move from one thought to another, making the patient's train of thought difficult to follow is classically described as *the knight's move*. This term comes from the game of chess where the knight is only allowed to move two squares forward and one to the side, or one forward and two to the side. A single word, rather than a line of thought may also set off abnormal associations as illustrated in the following examples:

(i)   'The far end of the ward got gold barred from me you see.'
(ii)   'Yes it looks like a red car to me. . . I don't know whether you'd say it was Redcar, near Whitby, Redcar. . . yes that's right. I can understand Yorkshire but I can't twig onto these youngsters at all.'

Even words with similar sounds can set off odd associations and where these occur they are called *clang associations*. For example one patient's speech contained the sequence 'astronaut, aster, aside'. Where both word and clang associations occur together in such rapidity that a series of words are spilled out without any apparent connection between them, the conglomeration is referred to as a *word salad*. Speech containing abnormal associations is often difficult to understand and is sometimes termed *incoherent*.

(*c*) *Neologisms*. These are completely new words, which may be built up from a number of other words. Sometimes the term describes the use of an accepted word which is used in an unusual way so it acquires a new meaning. 'Reichfact', 'Superbluous', and 'Disrefunct' are some examples we have heard patients using. In the following dialogue, a patient used six neologisms in the space of one sentence.

Nurse   'What's your opinion of this hospital?'
Patient   'Neglect.'
Nurse   'In what way?'
Patient   'In higher custody . . . and reproach of *minist* of beggary, of *disappearment* and *dismemberfying, disantchuting* in the eye of the *destrone* of the right *livmondont*.'

(*d*) *Thought interference*. Thoughts may be interrupted by hallucinations or other 'irrelevant' thoughts so that the patient finds it difficult to concentrate his thinking on the task in hand. With having so many thoughts at once the patient is unable to focus upon a given topic but may get caught up in all sorts of different ideas. He consequently has difficulty in keeping to the subject and his speech becomes *woolly* or *vague*. It becomes very difficult to follow, often going round in circles and appears to get nowhere and achieve nothing.

(*e*) *Derailment*. This disturbance can be viewed as the slide of speech from the original path to a new direction. The content of the new thought consists of ideas which lie close to the original train of thought, and so the patient's speech gradually moves away from the topic under discussion. One patient aptly described it as, 'Like a railway engine, running along a line, where someone else keeps changing the points'. This may lead the patient to excessive talking or *verbal diarrhoea* in trying to explain a particular point, as illustrated by a patient who took eight minutes of constant chatter to answer the question 'How are you today?'.

(*f*) *Concrete thinking*. This refers basically to thought which is bound or restricted to whatever we observe. Normally an individual can also think in abstract ways, being able to detach himself from the functional and practical properties of a present situation and consider it in relation to past events or future possibilities or other factors in the environment which do not have an obvious and immediate relation to whatever it is with which he is concerned. However, some patients seem to lack the ability to think in abstract ways. They will answer quite clearly concrete questions such as, 'How do you get to the canteen?', but more abstract ones cause the patient to give inappropriate answers. For example the question 'Why doesn't anyone live at Buckingham Palace?' was answered by a patient, 'My mother lives on the sun'. Consequently patients may also have difficulty in interpreting proverbs, confusing the literal and figurative meaning of words.

(*g*) *Other speech disturbances*. There are a few other forms of disturbance which do not fit easily into the above categories. Parts of thought, or grammatically necessary words may be dropped out or *omitted* so that the stream of thought is interrupted. For example, 'I and what is also so comic, consequently the nurse has not known me any more'. With *echolalia* a patient will repeat, often more than once, the last few words or syllables that another person has just said. Some patients use the same word to mean many different things, as where one patient called everyone, male or female, by the name Jean giving rise to statements like 'What do they call that Jean nurse?'

3. WILL (VOLITION)

There is frequently a loss of drive and lack of decision and determination among long-stay patients. This lack of initiative cannot wholly be attributed to the effects of a disturbance in psychological functioning however, for as we shall see the hospital environment itself can adversely affect a patient's behaviour in similar ways. The apathy and loss of energy seen in long-stay patients is most probably a result of a mixture

between the effects of his psychological condition and institutionalization. Often the behaviour associated with this disturbance in volition will
be solely attributed to the latter (institutionalization), but this is usually
not totally true. Some patients who have been in hospital for only a short
time will complain of a lack of energy and willpower. Further, a
reduction in drive may be apparent before admission to hospital, the
individual changing jobs, staying in bed all day and generally doing very
little at all. One patient said, 'What I found tiring at times was the effort
involved in making myself do things'. Some patients are therefore clearly
suffering from lack of willpower before their admission to hospital, but
this may worsen as a result of living in an institutionalized environment
for a number of years.

This lack of will is sometimes explained away by patients as the result
of interference by others on their decisions and actions. Where patients
complain of a loss of voluntary control over their thoughts, emotions and
actions, to the extent that they may feel they are being controlled by
electrical apparatus or earth satellites for example, they are said to be
showing *passivity feelings*.

4. EMOTION

Simply stated, an emotion is a state of arousal arising from physiological
changes which occur as a response to some event, and the type of
emotion we experience depends upon how we perceive the event. If we
perceive a situation as hostile we may interpret our arousal as anxiety.
We feel frightened. If we perceive the situation as enjoyable or cheerful
we may interpret the arousal as joy and feel happy.

Long-stay patients, especially those suffering with schizophrenia,
have been described as having a disturbance of emotion. Judging this,
however, is difficult for we only observe the outward expression of
emotion. It may be the case that while the person's 'emotions' remain
unaffected, the expression of them is disturbed. A patient may
accordingly 'feel' happy, or sad, but is unable to express it.

Recent research has examined emotion by alternative methods.
Instead of judging or evaluating the patient's expression of emotion,
patients have been asked to judge emotions such as joy and fear in
normal people. A great deal of evidence now suggests long-stay patients,
particularly chronic schizophrenic patients, are worse at recognising or
judging emotions in other people. It is as if the 'emotional world' is a
mystery to them. As we mentioned earlier, the long-stay patient has
enormous difficulty understanding other people, predicting how they
might react, judging how they feel and so forth. The patient's
psychological understanding of others is disturbed. This can take the
form of:

(a) *Flattening of affect.* Because the emotional world is meaningless or confused for the patient he may accordingly show a gross lack of emotional response. Facial expressions are often 'deadpan'. Patients may be unable or find it difficult to build up rapport with other people.

(b) *Inappropriate reactions.* The patient's emotional expressions, when they do occur, will often seem inappropriate because they arise from the patient's misinterpretation of the situation. Patients may thus seem insensitive, being coarse or brutal towards others, become excitable over slight incidents and maybe destroy clothes or furniture, or on occasions display what is called *incongruity* of emotion. This is where emotions are expressed which are quite out of keeping with the situation, possibly because they interpret the event differently from other people. For example, a patient may cry when a humorous story is told or talk of a child's death with a smile.

5. MOTOR BEHAVIOUR

Generally long-stay patients are inactive. When they move it is usually in a slow way, actions often appearing stiff and clumsy. This will most probably be as a result of the limited activity in which they are required to participate. When the majority of their time is spent sitting on the ward doing very little and they have engaged in this behaviour for years, it is hardly surprising they take proportionately longer to move from place to place. However, the physical actions of some patients may be disturbed in other ways:

(a) *Motor blocking.* This is similar to thought blocking, except that here a movement, though carried out correctly at first, stops abruptly before it is completed. For example, a patient dressing himself may come to an abrupt halt, unable to carry on for a period of time until prompted to do so. Alternatively, a patient may take a long time before an action is carried out in response to an instruction, as though there is a block between receiving the verbal instruction and performing the action. In this situation it is sometimes assumed that a patient is unable to carry out the request because of the long delay before anything happens, but patience is often rewarded by the patient complying with the request without further prompting.

(b) *Postures.* Where there is a complete lack of movement, with little if any reaction to external stimuli (as in catatonic patients), the state is called a *stupor.* Though this extreme state is rarely seen nowadays, some patients may maintain odd or bizarre postures for lengthy periods of time. For example, a patient may sit motionless staring at the floor, or turned away from ward activities. Sometimes a patient may stand with an arm in a rigid position or stare for long periods at a blank wall.

(c) *Mannerisms.* We all tend to have mannerisms such as tapping one's fingers or scratching one's head, but the mannerisms of long-stay patients seem to be different in form. The patient adopts gestures and poses common to other people but does so inappropriately or in an exaggerated or artificial way. Furthermore, the gestures or poses are usually peculiar to a given individual. For example, one patient always swayed three times before acting, another always walked round two tables before sitting down and yet another before each drink from a cup would stir the air above the cup with a spoon.

(d) *Stereotypy.* It is often difficult to distinguish this from mannerisms, but generally stereotypies refer to the constant repetition of any fixed sequence of behaviour. Some common examples of these include smacking of the lips, rubbing of the hands and rocking.

(e) *Other abnormal motor behaviours.* When a patient repeats the actions of someone else in the near vicinity this is known as *echopraxia,* and where the patient carries out every command given to him, even to the point of doing ridiculous things, this is called *automatic obedience.* Finally, *negativism* may be thought of as an active striving by the patient to defeat attempts to contact him. Thus, for example, when a visitor offers his hand the patient withdraws his own hand, or turns away.

Schizophrenia is the most common condition from which long-stay patients suffer. As such, the behaviour problems discussed in this chapter are certainly appropriate to them. However, none of the disturbances of functioning we have mentioned are exclusive to schizophrenia. Thus, for example, patients with head injuries may have hallucinations, and depressed patients show flattening of affect. What is important to remember is that a schizophrenic illness can manifest itself in all these ways—it is a remarkably multi-faceted disorder and, therefore, because the majority of patients on long-stay wards have had schizophrenic episodes, these are the behaviour problems we most frequently encounter.

By analysing behavioural problems in this way we hope to avoid the assumption that every patient who expresses a lack of emotion or a difficulty in concentrating is necessarily suffering from schizophrenia. It is often easy to fall into the trap of doing so, however, but it is far from helpful because the label itself might be completely wrong. Let us take, for example, an elderly patient who frequently thought other patients and staff on the ward were talking about him. His 'delusions of persecution' could easily have given him the label schizophrenic, but as it turned out he was simply suffering from the effects of ageing. His hearing had worsened over the years making it difficult for him to hear everything that was being said. Other people, such as staff discussing his medical condition, within his sight, could easily arouse the patient's suspicion as he was unable to pick out everything they were saying. Thus he could easily develop the notion of 'What are they saying about me?' Ageing is a process that frequently receives little attention but can have a number of effects on long-stay patients' behaviour.

Labelling also requires a type of judgement which for practical purposes tells us nothing. However, we *can* observe a patient's behaviour, and we *can* know in what way it is inappropriate or abnormal. We are concerned, therefore, not with the label tagged onto a patient, but with the problem behaviours he has. Once we shift our concern to behavioural problems, we are then in a position to begin treating what is wrong.

Chapter 2

THE ENVIRONMENTAL CONDITIONS

Environment refers to everything which occurs in the presence of a person. The many aspects of an environment can be roughly divided into the *physical* environment—those objects and tangible items which surround the person—and the *social* environment, created by the people who are present at any one time. Most people seek to avoid environments devoid of objects and/or people (e.g. prison cells, solitary confinement, or being 'sent to Coventry') because of the resulting lack of stimulation, as also they tend to avoid overstimulating environments (e.g. an extremely noisy room, or a shop crowded with people). Somewhere between these two extremes lies a 'preferred' situation. Whatever its nature an environment influences the way a person behaves.

Take, for example, the influence a social environment (a place of entertainment) has on our behaviour. We tend to sit quietly entering into little conversation with others at the cinema; clap, chant, shout and probably hurl abuse while watching a football game; or sing and dance at a 'pop' concert. Every environment promotes certain types of behaviour.

Patients, too, being sensitive to their surroundings, react and adapt to the particular environment in which they are functioning. Consequently, when a patient lives in one type of environment such as a long-stay ward for a number of years he is constantly faced with the same surroundings and predicaments which come to have a lasting effect on his behaviour. In this way a 'hospital environment' can create and maintain inappropriate behaviours which lead patients to depend eventually on the system. Russell Barton has called this process *institutionalization* and the behaviours which result form an *institutional neurosis.* He described this as being characterized by: 'Apathy, lack of initiative, loss of interest more marked in things and events not immediately personal or present, submissiveness, and sometimes no expression of feelings of resentment at harsh or unfair orders . . . a deterioration in personal habits, and a resigned acceptance that things will go on as they are . . . unchanging, inevitably and indefinitely.' (Russell Barton, 1976.)

13

Institutionalization is therefore a process distinct from the condition responsible for the person's admission to hospital, and it adds to the difficulties or problems the patient has. The severity of institutionalization varies from the one extreme of a very withdrawn patient who speaks little if at all, is shabbily dressed, sits in the same chair most of the day and every day, engages in no meaningful activity and needs continual prompting from nurses to perform even such basic actions as coming to meals. At the other extreme is the active patient who works well on or off the ward, is quite smart in appearance but whose dependence on the institution is apparent by his lack of desire or interest to leave the hospital.

Professor J. K. Wing suggests the degree of institutionalization is probably dependent on three factors:
1. The social environment
2. Individual susceptibility
3. Length of stay

1. *The social environment.* The individual learns to adapt to 'hospital life' and to processes operating in the hospital environment. These processes are discussed below. One might expect that the greater the severity of these processes, the greater would be the degree of institutionalization. The individual who spends years working at something which appears to be adaptive may, in fact, by adapting to a poor social environment over many years, be learning how to deteriorate.

2. *Individual susceptibility.* Some patients are more susceptible or sensitive to the effects of being in a hospital than others, and hence may show dependence on the institution and apathy about leaving, very soon after admission. Patients suffering from schizophrenia appear to be especially prone to institutionalization, which would seem to account for the fact that most long-stay patients have been or are suffering from this illness.

3. *Length of stay.* The longer a person has been exposed to a deadening monotonous routine, the more likely he is to show characteristic signs of institutionalization. This is reflected in discharge rates; the longer a patient stays in hospital the less likely he is to be discharged, and after two years of continuous hospitalization the chances of him leaving hospital drop suddenly. The difference between chronic and acute illness is made on this very dimension of time spent in hospital, a stay of two years usually being taken as the criterion that a patient has become chronic.

Unlike schizophrenia, where something 'internal', like thought processes or perceptions, appear not to be functioning normally, institutionalization is the result of 'external' processes in the environment operating on the patient. Institutionalized behaviour can be best understood, therefore, by examining these processes and how they work to affect behaviour adversely. These processes can be discussed under the following headings:

1. Admission
2. Loss of contact
3. Ward environment
4. Management of patients
5. Nurse–patient interaction

1. ADMISSION

Becoming a patient

When a person first enters hospital he usually experiences a number of traumatic events. In the psychiatric hospital, unlike other institutions such as prison and even the general hospital, there is no exact day for release. The average length of stay is about 6–8 weeks, but as there is no guarantee, the individual enters hospital without necessarily being able to see the light at the end of the tunnel. For some, admittedly a very few, it may be the start of a 15-, 20-, or 30-year 'stretch', and for a number of patients hospital is the place where they will spend the rest of their lives. A series of interviews and medicals with the doctor are followed by the bathing, weighing, listing of personal possessions, removal of valuables and assigning of a bed to the patient by the nurse—all of which has been aptly called a process of 'trimming' by Irving Goffman. That is, the individual is moulded into the role of 'patient' and is expected to behave like all other patients on the ward, complying with various rules and placing himself in the hands of those in charge of his treatment and care.

In the normal environment we relate to other people in a variety of ways. A male nurse in a hospital may, for example, act as a husband, a father, a gardener and darts player, in different and appropriate situations. However, a person, once admitted to hospital, always relates to people, in every aspect of his life, solely as a patient. He has but one role—that of the 'routinely pliant inmate'. He thus becomes recognized, not as an individual so much as by the symptoms which give him a diagnostic label, and by the tag of 'good', 'disruptive' or 'disturbed', depending upon how he behaves in his new role.

The new situation

The new patient, through his removal from the community, is also released from the stresses of ordinary life which may have contributed to his admission. He is relieved of economic responsibility and can avoid his work situation, where he may have had difficulty in coping with a complex job or in maintaining his rate of work. He is also removed from interpersonal family pressures which may have been distressing to him. The hospital in turn provides all the necessities of life. Food, bedding, clothing, warmth and money are available to all patients. Admission wards tend to be pleasantly furnished and facilities for recreation and leisure are generally quite good. Personal services, such as those of the chiropodist, dentist and hairdresser are provided, and in comparison with similar services available to people outside the hospital are often very prompt and extremely cheap, if not free.

While this situation has many advantages, one dangerous effect is of the hospital becoming a 'home' to some patients, which consequently lessens their motivation to leave. A patient may start to depend on the hospital for social recreation and company to such an extent that he becomes unwilling to venture out into the wider community. The binding effect that living in hospital can have was aptly described by one patient who said leaving the hospital was like 'the break-up of a good marriage'. Once a patient starts expressing a desire of not wanting to leave, or satisfaction with the way of life in hospital, institutionalization is taking a hold. When a patient is transferred to a long-stay ward, usually through lack of response to treatment, he faces many additional processes created by the new environment.

2. LOSS OF CONTACT

Social isolation

As we have seen, the mental condition a person is suffering from may cause the patient to withdraw into himself. Possibly as a way of protecting himself from overstimulation, or from distressing social relationships, he may reject contact with others. Interaction with those around him, including nurses, other patients and even his own visitors, becomes limited and he may shy away from activities which involve a social element, until he progressively becomes more and more socially isolated.

Restraint

Long-stay patients often have to seek permission before being allowed to leave the hospital grounds. As this may not be granted because of a variety of reasons, such as being seen as 'incapable' of looking after himself, or because of insufficient staff to go with him, his chances of contact with the community are reduced. If he wanders off without permission, he could be forcibly detained in the hospital. This is achieved by 'the locked door' approach, or by putting persistent absconders into dressing gowns.

Loss of visitors

Visitors may find it either physically difficult or unrewarding to visit because of:

Long distances. Many psychiatric hospitals are on the fringe of built-up areas, or may be many miles from the patient's home. Visiting may therefore be expensive, though visitors with low incomes can now receive special DHSS allowances; or inconvenient because of the amount of time it takes to travel to and from the hospital.

Poor facilities. Relatives and friends, though concerned and interested in a patient's welfare, may be discouraged from visiting a patient because of the poor facilities on the ward. Visitors may be 'put off' by the appearance and behaviour of other patients on the ward, by the lack of opportunity for private conversation, by the 'pestering' of other patients seeking cigarettes and lights and by the difficulty in obtaining some sort of refreshment. Also they may not be encouraged to write if their letters are not answered.

Patients, on the other hand, may be discouraged from visiting relatives because of the necessity of seeking permission and planning the visit, or because the relative does not want the patient at his home because of the stigma attached. Similarly a patient may find difficulty in writing letters because of the effort involved in obtaining the necessary materials from the nurse.

Hence over a period of time, and especially with placement on a long-stay ward, visits become less regular and less varied. That is, whereas initially a number of people would visit him, perhaps someone each day, after a number of years in hospital the visits gradually wane, so that the chronic patient might have one person visit him once a week or month (if he is lucky). The majority of chronic patients have very few visits at all, and many do not even have an annual Christmas or birthday visitor.

Provision of hospital facilities

In addition to providing the basic necessities and services, the hospital—more particularly in the past, but still today to some extent—provides many social and domestic facilities, thus reducing the patient's need to enter the community still further. As regards employment there may be, apart from occupational therapy and industrial therapy, work on the farm or garden, in the kitchen and workshops, or as a porter. For entertainment there are social evenings, dances, film shows, bingo sessions and facilities such as libraries, sports grounds and sports equipment. Because everything the patient needs can be provided within the institution, there is often little or no incentive to leave the hospital.

There are then a number of processes at work which combine to widen the gap between the patient's life and life in the community outside the hospital. The good amenities (on the admission ward) and facilities which remain available to the patient when transferred to a long-stay ward such as the chiropodist, hairdresser, socials and cinema may make the patient reluctant to leave hospital.

Then years of hospitalization with nobody writing or visiting, and little if any contact with life outside hospital leads the patient to live for the 'here and now'; to live one day at a time with little thought of getting out. The lack of outside involvement reduces the patient's chance of reacting in a normal environment and observing appropriate behaviour. He may consequently become unable to behave appropriately in the 'normal' environment where facilities change and new appliances emerge, for in the outside world time does not stand still (as it sometimes appears to in the institutionalized environment). Therefore, certain behaviours, such as those required in a supermarket or in catching a 'pay as you enter' bus, may be alien to him.

Having possibly lost his wife and friends, and being a 'stranger' in his own neighbourhood, the patient thus has few incentives to leave hospital and therefore is not motivated to re-enter the outside environment. Such an environment may conjure up fears of loneliness, an inability to adapt and lack of confidence to cope, which lead patients to rationalize their continued existence in the institution with comments like 'Leave me alone, Doctor, I'm not well enough to manage outside'.

3. WARD ENVIRONMENT

Many of the wards in which long-stay patients live are older, larger and populated with many more patients than is acceptable to modern thinking. This suggests that the physical and social environment of the ward may not be ideally suitable.

Physical surroundings

Though long-stay wards have undergone improvements in their physical surroundings most are still characteristically barren when compared to admission wards. They may now have curtains, plants and a few pictures, but most still have 'cold' bare walls of monotonous colour and lino-covered floors. Beds, chairs, lockers and other furniture are often similar in pattern, marked by cigarette burns and sometimes in need of repair. The level of noise may be disturbing and excessive, and though some noises such as telephone ringing are difficult to reduce in a ward situation, others such as constant loud television and/or radio sounds, slamming doors, and shouting from one end of the corridor to the other can be reduced with a little thought. Temperature and lighting arrangements may also not be ideal. Despite the efforts of domestic staff, inevitably a certain amount of dirt and rubbish accumulates. This can take the form of cigarette debris, sweet packets, the rubbish of persistent hoarders and unclean eating utensils.

Privacy

Although overcrowding is being reduced, patients may still need to share some facilities which are normally personal and private. Sleeping quarters, razors and sometimes clothes are examples of these. Two aspects of privacy which are normally cherished but which long-stay patients often have to do without are those of solitude and reserve.

Solitude is typically required in everyday life so that we can have time to ourselves for a while without being under constant observation. Solitude is sometimes difficult for patients to find when there are no single rooms or quiet rooms. Even the most private of places such as the toilets may have defective locks. Patients may therefore find places in the hospital gardens, shared by other patients, where they can withdraw temporarily from authority.

Reserve refers to a person's ability not to reveal certain aspects of himself which are particularly personal. Hospital wards are not always conducive to this, for nurses frequently know in detail the lives of their patients. Case notes need to be readily available for inspection, and the patient's behaviour and health may be matters for discussion in ward meetings. Though it may be necessary for doctor and nurses to know about the patient in some depth, the information should remain in the possession of those involved with the patient's treatment, confidentiality being especially important in preserving this state of the patient's privacy.

Other patients

The patient's companions being part of the environment in which he lives will, as such, influence his behaviour. He learns to live and adapt to the deadening existence as everyone else does, becoming indifferent to the events around him. As Leo Tolstoy said, 'There are no conditions to which a man cannot become accustomed, especially if he sees that all those around him live in the same way'. Patients may look dirty, bedraggled and unkempt, interact little between themselves and enter into little activity apart from searching for cigarette 'ends'. The patient who wants to engage in a sensible conversation, or an activity involving another person such as a game of cards, will find it difficult. Most patients entering such a ward soon lose interest and resign themselves to an inactive life shared with other patients, and thus a slide into the supine role of the long-stay patient, is made all the more likely.

Stimulation

The environmental poverty apparent from the lack of books, magazines, records and games often means time between meals is spent idly sitting around or mindlessly in front of the TV. There is little in the immediate environment to interest patients and what there is, in the form of games and hobbies, is usually kept under lock and key. Activities patients engage in are therefore mainly confined to duties relating to ward routine or their self care. Preparation for bed may start once tea has finished, so that most patients are in bed very soon after. The comments patients make when asked how they usually spend their time often reveal what little activity they engage in. 'I've nothing to do all day' or 'I just have to sit in the television room and watch time passing' are two examples.

The effect on patients of ward environments characterized by poor physical surroundings, the apathy of other patients and of understimulation is to increase what Professor Wing called the 'clinical poverty syndrome'. This 'syndrome' is typified by patients drawing away from people through cutting down their communication with them. Furthermore, there may be a fall off of patient's interests as such environments do not promote individual activities. Often a patient will not lose the ability to perform certain skills, but if the opportunities are not provided to practise them the skill becomes dormant.

4. MANAGEMENT OF PATIENTS

Herding

Many activities patients engage in are performed alongside other patients. For example, patients may have to share their sleeping area, wash alongside others in the washroom, file into the dining area, eat in overcrowded conditions, queue for medication, be shaved in sequence and herded into the living room to sit most of the day. The rationale behind this 'herding' approach is one of efficiency. If each patient does something completely different, a number of nurses are required to guide and supervise, and since nurses tend to be in short supply, managing patients in groups is more efficient. However, the nurses' role then becomes not so much one of guidance, but one of surveillance—seeing to it that everyone does what he has been told, under conditions where one person's misconduct is likely to stand out and hence be quickly rectified.

This conflict between humane standards and institutional efficiency is stretched to include even the personal possessions of the patient. Erving Goffman gives the following example of this conflict: 'The efficiency with which the clothes of patients can be kept clean is related to the fact that everyone's soiled clothing can be indiscriminately placed in a bundle, and laundered clothing can be redistributed, not according to ownership, but according to approximate size'. And sometimes it is very approximate!

The *personal possessions* patients bring with them into hospital may get lost, stolen or eventually wear out. Money and valuables are deposited in the hospital safe and may not be available to the patient at times convenient to him, particularly in the evening or weekends when the administrative staff are off duty. Soon patients come to own very few personal possessions, which may consequently lead to the collecting and hoarding of 'useless' items. The sort of basic items a long-stay patient may not personally own include:

1. A toothbrush, comb and clothes, and as a result he has little control over his own appearance. There may be little incentive for a patient to keep his clothes clean if there is no guarantee that he will wear the same ones next day.
2. Photographs of family, writing materials such as paper and pens, therefore finding it difficult to keep in contact with other people.
3. A locker with a key in which to keep personal belongings.

Both processes of herding and the gradual loss of possessions have a marked effect on the patient's behaviour. With the former the loss of individual freedom leads to a loss of events of personal significance for the patient. All the pleasant events which used to punctuate the patient's life and to which he used to look forward are lost. A Saturday night at the club, a week's holiday at the seaside, a friend's party or an anniversary simply become memories. Even his own birthday is often not recognized—in the institutionalized routine such personal events no longer occur.

Though the hospital tries to substitute for these events by giving Christmas presents, organizing holidays, day trips, dances and so on, they are of little personal significance. Because patients go *en masse* to these events little individuality can be fostered, and because the patient plays no part in organizing the events they have no personal value. Part of the pleasure an individual gains from an event is the involvement in planning and the excitement during the build up to the day of the event. Neither of these feelings is created for the patient since everything is planned for him, even down to the clothes he should wear.

With regard to his loss of possessions, the hospital again attempts to replace some items, and again these have usually no personal value since the patient has no choice in the matter. Unhappily these replacements tend to be of standard issue, they may have been previously used by another patient, may be prominently marked as belonging to the institution, and, especially in the case of clothing, may not fit properly. The patient's sense of individuality is thus at stake since he may soon become indistinguishable from other patients as far as clothing, haircut and so forth are concerned.

Staff arrangements

The most obvious characteristic of nursing administration is its hierarchial nature. The very clear system of authority means that any one of a particular staff grade can give orders to anyone of a lower grade. In practice this means that the patient, being bottom of the hierarchy, can be told what to do by any member of staff; and secondly that those having most patient contact are the nurses at the bottom of the hierachy, who also tend to be the least qualified.

Such a system breeds an authoritarian attitude, which Russell Barton suggested was revealed in many ways. For example, orders are often given in a dictatorial voice such as 'Sit down', 'I'll tell you when' and 'How many times have I told you. . . .' Patients may be shouted at across a ward and told off for minor infringements of the ward rules. The old system of medical superintendents in psychiatric hospitals undoubtedly encouraged authoritarianism, as the aim was usually to care for and control patients rather than provide treatment, since there was often little treatment available. Indeed nurses were trained to be authoritarian, since there was no other method of running the ward and relating to patients in which the superintendents could have equal confidence. Therefore, it is important not to blame staff but to remember that many older staff, and patients, initially learned their 'roles' under conditions which were sometimes grossly authoritarian. However, it is also important to consider that a new nurse, modelling herself on her superiors, can quickly fall into an authoritarian role.

The ease with which people fall into a role or social function is illustrated by an experiment with college students in America. They were asked to live out the role of either prison guard, or prisoner, in a specially built imitation prison. Dr Zimbardo, who conducted the experiment, had to bring it to a close after 5 days because 'guards' became too authoritarian and 'prisoners' too submissive. If this can happen to college students in 5 days, it is hardly surprising that patients exposed to an authoritarian regime for 20 years become *submissive,* accepting authority without question, sometimes to such an extent that they will carry out ridiculous tasks without question when told to do so.

The ward routine

Ward routines are intended to run so that procedures may be carried out with the minimum of fuss. They run smoothly where patients follow the system, which means there is always a danger that the patient is made to fit the system, rather than the system adapted to suit the individual's needs. By fitting in, the patient can easily become *passive,* offering little or no opposition to things done to him. Unco-operative patients disrupt the routine, and so they are made to conform either by what Goffman calls the privilege system or by punishment.

Staff may give patients privileges in exchange for obedience to their requests. Privileges may take many forms—having a more pleasant room or bed space, going off the ward without supervision, obtaining lights for cigarettes and generally being treated with extra kindness. These privileges and gratifications may be carved out of the flow of support and minor luxuries the patient had previously taken for granted. Because of the consequent lack of other opportunities for 'extras', the patient's attention can be wholly taken up with these minor privileges— searching for lights, cigarettes and cigarette-ends.

'Punishment' applied as a result of disrupting the routine may include suspension of privileges, such as moving a patient to a less desirable sleeping place, and may even extend to moving a patient to an undesirable ward.

5. NURSE–PATIENT INTERACTION

In recent years, the ways in which staff and patients interact with each other has been increasingly seen as one of the main aspects of institutionalization. It is difficult to generalize about the way in which these interactions take place, since they obviously depend on the individuals concerned, but three important effects tend to occur on long stay wards.

A general lack of interaction

Long-stay patients rarely talk among themselves. Even at mealtimes, which for most people is an opportunity to chat, patients talk to each other remarkably little. A stagnant routine, with little new or interesting to talk about, may contribute to this situation. The nurse, who may be the only contact a patient has with the changing world outside, has 30 patients to look after and may not have time to sit and talk. Indeed, the nurse's whole approach may be directed towards keeping the ward tidy, clean and quiet, as it often has been in the past, rather than cultivating a therapeutic atmosphere and emphasizing the importance of relationships with patients. Without meaningful interaction with others, patients remain *socially withdrawn.*

Nurses do things for patients

Patients are often denied the opportunity to do things because the nurse finds it quicker to do them herself. Hence making beds, shaving, washing, dressing, making drinks and even feeding are often done for patients by the nurse. This gives patients ample opportunity to become idle. Furthermore, the patient's dignity may be at stake, for although he may be capable of performing these actions, he is just never given the chance.

The elementary decisions a person normally has to make in his day-to-day existence may also be denied the person in hospital. Nurses show a tendency to decide for the patient which clothes and shoes to wear, when to go to the hairdressers, which bed to sleep in, where to sit at mealtimes, when to go out, and so on. Sometimes quite fundamental decisions such as a change of physical treatment or a move to another ward are made for the patient without his involvement in the decision making, and often he may be the last one to know of the decision.

The patient's ability to make decisions is gradually eroded away, because he is no longer required to think things out. This leads to a *lack of initiative*, where the patient increasingly needs to be prompted into action, lacking the ability to act spontaneously and control his own behaviour, since almost all decisions regarding the circumstances of his life are made for him.

Nurses pay attention to undesirable behaviour

It is easy to think of the individual who sits inactive most of the day, who comes for his meals when called, is obedient to orders, and who causes no trouble to the staff through asking, for example, for extra leave or clean clothes as the 'good' patient. Such behaviour can therefore be encouraged, perhaps quite unwittingly; but as we have seen it can lead to the patients becoming passive and lacking in initiative.

There may be a notion among staff that if a person is in a mental hospital he must be sick, or abnormal in some way—otherwise, why would he be there? Hence abnormality becomes both accepted and expected. Undesirable behaviour may be tolerated because of a 'He can't help it' attitude, and any unusual request or idiosyncratic behaviour portrayed by the patient is regarded as evidence of mental disorder, so confirming the patient's illness. Thus an individual who occasionally shouts at others may in the community as a whole be regarded as showing acceptable or at least tolerable traits of asserting authority or responding to frustration, but in hospital he will probably be labelled aggressive and be prescribed drugs to calm him down.

The amount of time a nurse spends with an individual patient is dependent to some extent upon how much undesirable behaviour is shown. We have seen how the nurse 'does' for those patients who cannot dress, shave and so on, but she must also be on hand to quell any disruptive behaviour such as aggression and destruction of property. We therefore see that the nurse gives a great deal of her time and attention to patients who show undesirable behaviour, and perhaps very little time to those whose behaviour is acceptable or normal. Thus patients may learn that they can gain attention quite effectively by behaving in undesirable ways. On wards where there are few nurses and thus little individual attention, the patient may find the only way to secure an interaction with a nurse is by being disruptive. Odd speech, because of its novelty or unusual quality may be encouraged if nurses listen or laugh, and as the patient may feel 'secure' if he can please staff, this type of behaviour will increase. In long-stay wards, therefore, normal behaviour may be rarely noticed or attended to, whereas inappropriate behaviour may be the patient's key to obtaining time and attention from nurses.

Physical disabilities

Long-stay patients not infrequently have some physical disability which is not directly due to their psychiatric condition. Many chronic patients have a raised pain threshold, so they may not complain of a problem until well beyond the point where a normal person would seek medical attention.

On the other hand, other patients' complaints may be disregarded because they are believed to be delusional. One patient, for example, complained of weak legs and said this was due to another patient taking her blood. However, on examination she was found to have anaemia, which had affected the spinal nerves and caused wastage of muscle in one leg.

Other common physical problems, though perhaps not so severe, involve sensory loss. One patient had been diagnosed as 'subnormal', and had lived in a hospital for the mentally handicapped for years before transfer to a psychiatric hospital. An examination revealed that her ears were impacted with wax, causing an apparent deafness which in itself had led to part of her dullness. Removal of the wax resulted in social improvement, despite some continued hearing loss. Similarly, many patients have bad eyesight, a natural consequence of ageing. On one ward up to 80% of patients required spectacles, revealed initially by careful observation by nurses. During group treatment sessions the problem became apparent through the patients' inability to thread needles, and their stumbling attempts at reading. Solution of such problems, through prescribing hearing aids and spectacles, can only be successful if the patients are trained to use them properly. Similarly provision of dentures is a waste of time if the patient is not guided and supervised in using them properly.

In this chapter, an attempt has been made to outline some of the factors that lead to institutionalized behaviour. These factors all interact with each other in any one ward to produce a pattern that may be highly distinctive of separate wards in any one institution. Environments characterized by such factors lead to certain types of behaviour. The most common are:

Loss of motivation	No desire to leave hospital. No plans for the future.
Lack of initiative	The inability of patients to make decisions and control their own behaviour.
Lack of interest	Interests are restricted to the satisfaction of a few immediate needs, rather than including events and people not in the immediate environment.

Apathy	A reluctance to become involved in events around them.
Submission	Uncomplaining and unquestioning acceptance of authority.
Loss of individuality	A loss of distinct and unique characteristics.
Deterioration in personal habits	Losing the capacity to care for personal appearance, hygiene and grooming.

Chapter 3

TRADITIONAL TREATMENT

We can chart our future clearly and wisely only when we know the path which has led to the present. ADLAI STEVENSON (1952)

Today, it is hard to believe some of the ways people with 'mental disorders' were treated in the early part of the nineteenth century, when most of the large psychiatric hospitals were opened. Some of the records of mechanized restraint portray horrifying scenes of patients being chained up for several years with only very limited movement.

Many of the 'treatments' which were used to promote recovery during the nineteenth century now appear bizarre and brutal, though a certain degree of success was attributed at the time to these methods. Bleeding and purging were early treatments considered acceptable, though many patients nearly bled to death. The revolving chair was another form of treatment, where the patient was strapped to a chair and spun round at about one hundred revolutions per minute. Restraint took the form of straps securing a patient to a chair or bed, leather or steel handcuffs, strait-waistcoats, and muzzles to prevent patients biting other people. Seclusion was considered beneficial in certain cases until quite recently.

Despite little progress as regards treatment during the nineteenth century, efforts were made to improve the patient's diet, hygiene, accommodation and pastimes. Employment began to be thought of as beneficial, and only recently has work within the hospital on routine domestic tasks been frowned upon. Allegations that such work was 'cheap' labour resulted in shift of emphasis from the performance of such duties towards occupational therapy, art therapy and, more recently, industrial therapy.

Many of the treatments used throughout the nineteenth century helped in maintaining quite a high rate of recovery despite their 'barbaric' nature. However, each treatment method in turn fell into disuse, not necessarily because of a lack of effectiveness but because popularity would begin to be focused on a more fashionable method. Thus 'out of date' methods would fade into the historic pages of psychiatric textbooks.

27

Many of the criticisms levelled at these earlier treatments can also be applied to the techniques developed in the twentieth century. Two of particular interest are that:

1. Many treatment methods were discovered almost by accident or on a 'hunch' that a certain technique may be beneficial, and thus there was no theoretical basis or understanding of why they worked.
2. Many treatments have had disastrous effects on some patients. They have degraded and at times physically injured patients. Many present-day patients, especially those who have been hospitalized for a number of years, have been recipients of early twentieth-century treatments and suffered some side-effects as a result.

The twentieth century has brought a new spate of physical treatments, the main ones of concern being:

1. Insulin therapy
2. Leucotomy
3. Electroconvulsive therapy (ECT)
4. Drug therapy

1. INSULIN THERAPY

This was introduced in 1935 by Sakel, initially for improving the physical and mental state in cases of severe anorexia. He was then encouraged to try the method on schizophrenic patients. It involved the giving of insulin in the correct dosage to induce a coma; a technique requiring great medical and nursing skill. The patient would then be resuscitated, and the whole procedure repeated daily for a variable number of weeks, dependent on the patient's response. Although a number of remarkable recoveries were documented, 22 years after the treatment had been first used, it was demonstrated by Ackner and colleagues that the insulin itself was of no therapeutic value in the treatment of schizophrenia. Rather any benefit gained by the patient was through associated variables such as the complete rest, the company of other patients, the ample meals provided after the treatment, the playing of games with nurses and the great deal of attention given by doctors and nurses involved in the treatment. The method thus fell into disuse in the treatment of schizophrenia, though a modified form of insulin therapy is used nowadays in stimulating appetite. However, the failure did bring a new realization that enthusiasm, a hopeful attitude and good nursing were in themselves beneficial.

2. LEUCOTOMY (or lobectomy)

This treatment originated from a hypothesis that certain mental illnesses were possibly due to a disorder of the nervous system within the brain whereby abnormal patterns of impulses travelled along particular pathways which interfered with normal responding. In the hope of interrupting these pathways, and thus reducing disturbed behaviour, the main white fibre connections to the frontal lobes of the brain were severed. In the 1950s the operation was performed on many long-stay patients, and though some did improve sufficiently to leave hospital, a large number remained. The irreparable brain damage often left patients with various side-effects such as blunting of emotion, lack of volition and stuttering. Though the techniques have become more sophisticated so that more selected areas can be cut or ablated, the operation is now rarely considered to be of any benefit for long-stay schizophrenic patients.

3. ELECTROCONVULSIVE THERAPY (ECT)

Based on the now false belief that schizophrenia was rare in epileptics, Cherletti and Bini suggested that the induction of epileptic seizures in schizophrenic patients might prove beneficial. Originally convulsions were drug-induced, but nowadays the method consists of passing a high-voltage electric current through the brain by means of electrodes placed on the head. Originally this was given 'straight'—that is, without anaesthetic and must have been a terrifying experience for the patient, held down by body straps and the hands of many nurses. Nowadays an anaesthetic and muscle relaxants are given prior to the induction of electric shock. The details of what exactly happens during this treatment remains uncertain, but the induced fit is presumed responsible for any therapeutic effect. Many psychiatrists and nurses are staunch believers in its value, but there have been very few controlled studies to show that any benefit gained by patients is actually due to the shock. One experiment, for example, showed that simply anaesthetizing patients when they believed they were to have the shock, but who did not, also helped them to improve. This again suggests that associated factors such as increased nurse attention, and the patient's expectancy of improvement may be of equally beneficial value.

Such an effect is often termed a *placebo* effect. When a person undergoes treatment, improvement in behaviour may often occur because the individual simply expects to improve since he believes he is being treated. The agents bringing about improvement may then be the factors associated with the 'treatment', such as increased attention, expectancy and the therapeutic milieu which the patient is in, rather than the treatment method itself.

4. DRUG TREATMENT

Some of the older drugs such as barbiturates and paraldehyde which were used to calm down or sedate patients, are rarely used today because they often caused confusional states. Since the introduction of tranquillizing drugs in 1952, phenothiazines have been the most widespread form of treatment for schizophrenic patients. Chlorpromazine (Largactil) is the most frequently used. Tranquillizers, in contrast to the overall dampening effect of sedatives, work selectively on the emotional and motor functions, leaving thinking processes and memory largely unaffected. Hence, in therapeutic doses, tranquillizers cause no impairment in level of awareness, but reduce levels of inappropriate emotional and motor behaviour. This enables the patient to regain a measure of control over his behaviour, making him more amenable to other forms of treatment, and thereby increasing the chances of developing adaptive coping responses.

Tranquillizers have had a tremendous effect on the behaviour of schizophrenic patients, especially in the acute stages of illness, but also in reducing inappropriate behaviour of the chronic patient to manageable levels. Tranquillizers also have certain advantages which contribute to their preference over other types of treatment. These include: *ease of administration*—more patients can be treated more efficiently and economically; *speed of action*—change in behaviour can be rapidly brought about; *rapid evaluation*—any detrimental effects can be readily reversed; and *flexibility*—dosages can be readily changed and drugs can be used in combination with other drugs.

The effectiveness of a drug in changing behaviour, however, is influenced by a number of factors. Two factors of particular concern are:

(*a*) *The patient's state.* As each patient and the problems he presents are unique, predicting the nature and extent of response to any drug is a difficult business. This explains why often a few drugs have to be tried in different dosages and different combinations before a successful formula is found.

(*b*) *The patient's expectations.* When ill, we all expect to improve if we take a prescribed tablet. The act of tablet taking is seen by patients as treatment. Studies substituting placebo tablets (tablets which are chemically neutral) indicate that between a half and two-thirds of long-stay patients, especially those on low dosages, may not require active medication. This again indicates the effect of other variables in the treatment situation which are maintaining behaviour, and poses the question of how many patients are on maintenance doses when they need not be. This is especially important when tranquillizers may produce various side-effects such as skin sensitivity, limb tremors, thirstiness and possible liver damage.

As well as side-effects, drug treatment may well have other disadvantages. Patients may fail to take tablets, but the recent introduction of long-acting drugs given by intramuscular injection reduces this possibility. Secondly, excessive usage of a drug in an attempt to manage patients may give rise to drowsiness and apathy, and liberal dosages of night sedation may lead to incontinence. Furthermore, the long-term effects of certain drugs is still largely unknown. Drugs reduce most of the disturbing symptoms, but fail to affect the basic pathological processes. This is often observed when a drug is removed, the patient frequently reverting to his previous disturbing level of behaviour. Drugs therefore are not 'cures' and, as such, are not sufficient on their own—other means of treatment are needed to enable the long-stay patient to function again at an appropriate level. This has for a long time been supplied in the form of various hospital departments such as industrial and occupational therapy, and more recently by the development of therapies based on psychological principles.

There are a number of important points to be drawn from our discussion of physical treatments with regard to long-stay patients. We have previously mentioned that most of the treatments have little if any theoretical basis, that the possibility of damaging side-effects is very real. In addition we see:

(a) The social factors associated with the treatment regime seem to have contributed in no small way to the patient's improvement. There are numerous variables in any treatment which appear common to all treatment situations: *novelty*—anything new creates interest and enthusiasm in staff and patients alike; *attention*—any treatment usually results in more attention being paid to individual patients and their problems; and *expectation*—patients may expect and are expected to improve if something called treatment is going on. Results of treatment may owe more to these associated social factors, than to the theoretical correctness of the therapeutic procedures used. Patients may benefit therefore if these social factors can be harnessed and developed as treatment agents themselves.

(b) Physical treatments have followed the traditional 'medical model' approach of diagnosis, treatment and cure. The nurse has thus adopted a caring role, providing for patients' physical welfare. However, for the chronic patients resident on long-stay wards, this approach has failed to work. Patients have been diagnosed and prescribed treatment but they have not been 'cured'. Doctors trained in this approach who find patients failing to respond may continue to apply the medical model, though it fails to work. Thus more and more drastic treatments are prescribed until 'as a last resort' a leucotomy may be performed.

There are alternatives to physical treatments which avoid these criticisms—psychological treatments. There are many psycho-therapeutic techniques, but one of particular interest to us, because of its applicability to long-stay patients is that of behavioural treatment (sometimes called behavioural psychotherapy, behaviour modification or behaviour therapy).

Following a behavioural treatment approach 'odd' behaviours are not regarded as symptoms of an underlying illness (as with a medical model), but as behaviours which are inappropriate for normal social existence, and which therefore require modification. Behaviour therapists may even argue that there is some continuity between normal and abnormal states, but that the balance has been tipped in the direction of abnormality by the sufferer's history of learning. Behaviour modification differs from other treatments in terms of its reliance upon the principles of learning theory. If a patient's speech is unacceptable, for example, then the aim of behavioural treatment is to modify the patient's words and sentences—he is taught to speak appropriately. As Schaefer and Martin say, behaviour modification essentially 'concentrates on developing or reinstating behaviours which are necessary for effective functioning in a social context'.

There are a number of techniques based on learning principles and which therefore come under the rubric of behaviour therapy. These include systematic desensitization, flooding and aversive conditioning which are used most effectively to help in the treatment of acute patients' problems. With long-stay patients, the most appropriate form of behavioural treatment is *operant conditioning,* a technique formulated by Professor Skinner, an American psychologist. The central proposition is that the consequences which follow a particular piece of behaviour influence the future occurrence of that behaviour. Basically, behaviours which are followed by desirable consequences (reinforcers) increase or are maintained, while those followed by undesirable consequences (no reinforcement or punishment) diminish. Structuring the patient's environment so that appropriate behaviour is followed by desirable consequences and inappropriate behaviour by undesirable consequences has led to improvement in a number of behaviours, such as social withdrawal, mutism and incontinence. This is very much a simplification but sufficient for a basic understanding of the procedures involved in behaviour modification. We will of course be looking at the theory and the practical methods of relevance to treatment of the long-stay patient in much more detail in the following chapters.

Behaviour modification does not suffer from the criticism of lacking a theoretical basis as many of the physical treatments do. The evidence upon which the theories behind behavioural therapy were built have generally been carefully and painstakingly collected under controlled experimental conditions. Thus behavioural treatment, or the learning approach, appears to be more scientific, and this therefore enables us to have confidence in using the procedures. In general, the theories underlying behavioural treatment are properly constructed and are able to be tested by direct experiment.

A further criticism of physical treatments was the possibility of enduring side-effects. Because behavioural treatments focus directly on the problematic behaviour and since its methods are derived from well-established 'laws of learning', we are able to predict with much more certainty the results of treatment. Side-effects will only occur as a result of the techniques being used wrongly. Much care needs to be taken with techniques such as punishment, and where such care and consideration is absent, undesirable effects can and will result. Careless and haphazard use of procedures may produce changes in behaviour, but these will tend not to be in the desired direction and therefore it becomes inappropriate to consider the techniques as behavioural 'treatment'. Where techniques are used appropriately, desirable changes in behaviour can be achieved reliably, efficiently and with some degree of certainty.

The final criticism of physical treatments was the lack of controlled experimental studies to discover whether it is the treatment agent itself or the associated social factors (e.g. extra attention and expectancy) which are of major therapeutic value. Behavioural treatment emphasizes the importance of these social elements, as they are often systematically utilized as therapeutic tools around which a treatment programme is designed.

Behavioural treatment has generally been conducted in sessions with one patient and a therapist (usually a psychologist). The therapist may attempt, for example, to modify a patient's bizarre speech by reinforcing appropriate speech and not reinforcing bizarre or delusional speech. However, the constraints of only one therapist conducting treatment, and the small number of sessions which can be given each week, limit the patient's time in treatment and hence its effectiveness.

By making the environment in which the patient lives a treatment area, the patient can be treated every hour of the day, often as a member of a group of patients, and not by just a single therapist but by all the people involved in his life. This includes nurses, who become most important in the patient's rehabilitation, not by maintaining their traditional 'caring' role but by developing their ability to interact therapeutically with patients.

Patients are helped to modify their 'odd' responses by teaching them to develop their social skills during participation in varied group experiences. David Clark has termed programmes which aim to modify behaviour by making the patient's environment a treatment area *social therapy*. He suggests that effective social therapy programmes include; *activity*—'almost any activity is good, but purposeful, socially valued, rehabilitative activity is best'. Professor Wing found during an 8-year study that it was those patients who were active (in ward work, industrial and occupational therapy) who showed the greatest advances; *freedom* —allowing the patient freedom of choice and providing opportunities which involve decision making on the part of the patient; *responsibility* —giving patients back their independence so they are encouraged to use their own initiative again. Social therapies are characterized by increased social interaction between staff and patients, by the participation of patients in a number of different activities, and by an exposure of the patient to a variety of social settings. Two interesting developments in this field are:

1. The therapeutic community.
2. The token economy

1. THE THERAPEUTIC COMMUNITY

Maxwell Jones is the main exponent of this form of treatment. Both staff and patients work together in an attempt to increase the individual's awareness and understanding of what he is doing to himself and other people. Daily meetings are held to discuss matters of general interest to the community and debate the setting up of new rules or regulations where necessary. Patients have equally as much say in the running of the ward as staff and often chair the meetings. During the rest of the day workshops, domestic groups, discussion groups and so forth meet to analyse what is happening among the members of the group at that time.

There are relatively few therapeutic communities functioning in Britain at the present time, probably because of the scepticism and hostility people have towards them. Many nurses feel threatened by this form of approach for it deprives them of their traditional role but does not replace this deprivation with a role they can readily identify with. There may also be doubts about the efficiency of the method and apprehension about inevitable effects such as tolerance of antisocial behaviour, accumulation of dirt and apparent disorder.

2. THE TOKEN ECONOMY

This method of treatment provides a structure for the practice of behavioural treatment to a whole group of resident chronic patients. The idea was first developed by two American psychologists, Ayllon and Azrin in the early 1960s. Basically, specific aims for the ward are laid down, and each patient has specific goals of his own. Progress towards these goals is systematically rewarded with tokens by the nursing staff. The patient then exchanges the tokens he has earned for items he may want, such as cigarettes, a single room or an extra half-hour in bed in the morning.

There are many variations on this basic theme and wards develop their own particular styles in response to the problems which are prevalent. Research work performed so far shows that token economies can help patients improve in a number of areas of behaviour, sometimes to a level of improvement whereby they can be discharged back into the community. An interesting finding is that it is not so much the token which produces improvement, but the social elements which go with the giving of a token—such as praise, attention and feedback to the patient on how well he has done—which may constitute the vital therapeutic factor. This finding corresponds with the findings of the earlier treatments we reviewed. However, behavioural treatments, in contrast to treatments based on the medical model, emphasize, utilize and structure these social factors and so enhance 'the placebo effect' in a way which can be of maximum benefit to the long-stay patient.

The recent emergence of behavioural treatment has given hope to those patients who otherwise might have remained fixtures in the long-stay wards. There is no doubt such patients have benefited from the introduction of phenothiazine drugs but their effect is more one of reducing bizarre behaviours rather than of building up social skills. The most effective attempts at rehabilitating long-stay patients will therefore come from a combination of drug therapy, modifications to the patients' environment and treatment of specific problems with techniques derived from behaviour modification.

SECTION II
THE NURSE AS THERAPIST

Chapter 4

REHABILITATION

Rehabilitation is a familiar word to doctors, nurses, remedial gymnasts, occupational therapists, and all people employed in the 'caring' services. Though all may declare their main aim to be rehabilitation of their patients, the way each one would define it could differ considerably; not only between each professional group, but also between members of the same group.

There are two main areas of controversy concerning the meaning of rehabilitation:

1. One school of thought makes a distinction between rehabilitation and treatment, regarding them as separate entities with different goals, but which are, nevertheless, complementary to each other. Another group considers rehabilitation and treatment as parts of the same process.
2. An opinion held by some people is that the term 'rehabilitation' should be confined solely to those patients being prepared for discharge from hospital. It is a view contested by others.

Rehabilitation and treatment

Many people understand rehabilitation to mean, 'the activities which prepare patients to take their place in the community *after* medical treatment has been completed'. In psychiatric hospitals these treatments consist mainly of a course of drugs, electric convulsive treatment and, occasionally, non-medical treatment such as individual or group psychotherapy. The follow-up activities, designed to prepare patients for life outside the hospital, are understood to involve training in work and domestic skills, as well as education in the knowledge and use of the facilities available in the community.

On the other hand some people regard rehabilitation as a single continuing process and do not make any distinction between medical treatment and the training activities which follow. They declare that rehabilitation starts the very moment a patient enters hospital and may continue even after he has been discharged from hospital.

An example of this continuing process can be seen in the role of the community nurse, who may be engaged in making regular visits to a patient's home, long after his discharge from hospital. The purpose of the community nurse's visit may be to administer to the patient his regular maintenance dosage of drugs via intramuscular injections. It may also include counselling the patient, monitoring his behaviour and reporting all observations to the appropriate member of her team. According to this concept, 'rehabilitation' never ends.

Rehabilitation—the patients to whom it applies

Opinions may differ when deciding the limits of the boundary to which the term 'rehabilitation' should apply.

Some say the word 'rehabilitation' should be confined to those patients undergoing treatment or training who have been assessed as having the potential to live and maintain themselves in the community. Others are convinced the boundaries of the term 'rehabilitation' should be extended, in order to include patients undergoing treatment or training who, though not regarded as capable of ever living outside hospital, have the potential to improve and maintain their improvement, with minimal supervision, within the hospital.

When a patient is receiving treatment, or training, from a number of therapists at different times, one thing is important; whatever definition of 'rehabilitation' is chosen, it must be one agreed to by all the therapists concerned. A co-ordinated approach to the patient is essential in order to plan treatment and assess achievement of identifiable goals. Without this unity of purpose, well-meaning services of the specialist groups become fragmented, produce ill-feeling between the disciplines, confuse the patient and decrease the chance of a successful outcome of any form of rehabilitation.

The era of multi-disciplinary teams in the health service has arrived. They are an essential and practical concept, for no single therapist can provide all the forms of treatment which may be required by a patient from his admission to his discharge from hospital.

If multi-disciplinary teams are to function efficiently, the members of each team must not confine themselves to discussions at committee meetings, but start to operate and co-operate practically at ward level— the place where all therapy begins in hospitals. A unifying approach to treatment for health teams to consider is that of behavioural modification. Without doubt the key members of any team at ward level are nurses. With the knowledge, practice and experience of behavioural modification techniques, nurses can become very valuable and skilled members of the rehabilitation team.

WHAT IS REHABILITATION?

Rehabilitation, in our view, is a word which describes an active process in which at least two people are involved; the person with a disability (the patient), and a helper (the therapist).

To rehabilitate means: to re-establish
to reconstruct
to reinstate
to renew
to regain

All these terms indicate that rehabilitation is a building activity which attempts to: 'Restore a person's physical and mental capacities and improve the quality of his life to a level which is, as near as possible, to that which existed prior to his illness'.

The way this can be achieved is called *therapy* and therapy means 'treatment to heal'.

A commonly used phrase is often quoted by people suffering from some form of psychological stress: 'I feel shattered—my nerves have gone to pieces', they say. Their family and friends may describe the sufferer's state as a 'breakdown', and advice directed to the sufferer is usually: 'Try to pull yourself together'.

This feeling of disintegration and depersonalization is quite common to those suffering from various forms of psychological disorder. It is particularly severe in certain forms of schizophrenia. The advice 'Pull yourself together', is, of course, a hope rather than a practical action the victim can perform. It does, however, clearly identify the goal of treatment.

If *therapy* means 'treatment', and to heal is 'to make whole', then the aim of treatment is to help to 'pull the person together'—to make him whole—in other words to restore him to health.

A *therapist* is one who conducts treatment, has detailed knowledge of the particular discipline he practises, has acquired skills in the use of procedures and techniques, is able to establish a good relationship with patients being treated, is aware of potential problems which may arise and is also aware of the limitations of the form of treatment as well as its benefits.

One can never be certain that a particular treatment will be successful. Therefore, rehabilitation involves hope and confidence in the treatment.

A general air of optimism that the treatment will have a beneficial effect on the patient may be the only way the therapist can involve the patient and motivate him to become an active participant in his own treatment. From the moment a patient first enters the admission ward of a psychiatric hospital, he receives a great deal of attention from a variety of people. The psychiatrist interviews and gives him a physical examination, the nurses attend to his needs and comforts, laboratory technicians take blood samples and the patient may be taken on a trip to visit the X-ray department of the hospital. All these events happen within the first few days of admission, when the patient is under the greatest stress.

Despite his torment and despondency, a patient may often sense his pessimism may not be justified, for there are people around him making some attempt to help him; people with experience of treating similar conditions to his own. Surely they would not initiate treatment if they thought he could not be helped?

While in hospital, and during the course of physical treatment, the patient may meet the social worker who will attend to his economic and family problems which may allay his anxiety and prepare the way for his return home. The occupational therapist will provide him with useful activities which may enable him to regain interest in his environment. Relatives and friends will regularly appear at visiting periods and maintain his links with his family and news of local events in the community. He will, most likely, be able to return home in a relatively short time.

Within average time span of 6–8 weeks after treatment, many patients may be expected to have recovered to a level of health sufficient to justify their discharge from hospital and to return to their own home. Though it may be true that some patients will return to hospital after a year or so— some even within a few months of discharge—a similar treatment and period of time in hospital may be all that is required for them to return once more to their home.

The patients who do not respond favourably to the available treatments may eventually be transferred to the long-stay wards. Indeed if a patient has no visiting family or friends, does not have suitable living accommodation in the community and is considered by the doctor to be incapable of looking after himself, his transfer to a long-stay ward will be inevitable. After all, an admission ward is a rehabilitation area.

Rehabilitation areas require a flow of movement of patients into and out of such wards. The only way to achieve this flow is to be able to balance admissions with discharges. A danger to this system is the patients who do not improve with treatment and who therefore 'block' the system. If a patient is unfit to be discharged from hospital the only solution is to find an area within the hospital to which he can be transferred. In this way the small wards containing chronic patients have developed into large wards with their consequent problems of institutionalization. Once a patient becomes a resident in a long-stay ward, his personal situation changes. From being the centre of the attention of many therapists and receiving active treatments, he changes to being one of a group of many patients who are receiving 'passive' treatments—that is, treatments which involve taking drugs to contain problems rather than reduce or extinguish them. No longer do social workers and doctors visit or interview him with such regularity. The previous prevailing mood of optimism, experienced on the admission ward, wanes as the interest of the therapists diminishes.

Nurses on the long-stay ward read the patient's case notes and can often see words such as 'poor' and 'hopeless' to describe a patient's prognosis. If the psychiatrist's forecast of the course of the patient's illness is so pessimistic, who are nurses to say otherwise? This rational conclusion results in the nursing staff adopting a 'caring' attitude to the patient, for if the patient cannot be expected to improve, the only humanitarian thing to do is to 'look after' him.

Patients who arrive on the long-stay wards are 'failures'. Those who have been diagnosed as suffering from 'schizophrenia' are particularly likely to regard themselves as failures, for their disorder will have frequently developed between 14 and 20 years of age, the periods when achievements at school and work are evaluated.

School reports probably described the scholar as 'silly', 'lazy', and 'lacking in concentration'. Employers probably regarded their employee as 'unreliable', 'inefficient', 'never punctual'. Their employment history is often one of frequent changes of job which lasted for only brief periods. Failure follows them into hospital and, when they do not improve with treatment, their failure may be regarded as complete when they enter a long-stay ward.

If relatives at any time enquire about the patient's progress, the answer will usually be 'not much change'. If they desire to know his chances of discharge, the non-committal response of nurses is often sufficient answer to their questions.

Sometime between admission to the hospital and after a lengthy residence on the long-stay ward, the florid signs of many psychiatric disorders appear to subside. Their disruptive and odd behaviours become reduced, and such patients are often referred to as 'burnt-out' schizophrenics. There may well be a need, at this point of their illness, to reassess them with a view to treating their remaining behaviour problems.

The concept of a rehabilitation area for long-term patients in hospital is not impossible. Many hospitals have developed such areas and reversed the trend of 'gloom and doom' prevalent among many nurses working on these wards as well as the patients living on them. Inevitably, the concentration of attention has been on the higher level patients, and the goal of treatment has been 'discharge from hospital' to hostels, group homes and the occasional success of private accommodation. Eventually, the high level patients are 'creamed off'.

There is, however, another group of patients whose chances of living in the community are poor, but who could, with some form of behavioural treatment, become more independent of the nursing staff and have a better quality of life. These patients represent the majority of long-term residents and active treatments are also possible for them. The target for their rehabilitation is a more modest one; that of leading a more independent life within the hospital. Rehabilitation must, therefore, include the provision of a suitable environment which, hopefully, will maintain improved behaviours.

Treatment and hope are linked together. Rehabilitation is for long-term patients as well as short-stay patients. The flow of movement of patients entering the long-stay wards must balance with the patients being discharged out of hospital to group homes and hostels in the community. For those patients who are unable to live in the community, areas in the hospital need to be upgraded in structure and amenities to maintain the behaviours which have improved with treatment. It is to these areas such patients should be transferred.

There is no reason why there should be any difference between an admission ward and a long-term ward in a psychiatric hospital other than the length of stay of the patient during treatment.

Chapter 5

MODIFYING THE ENVIRONMENT

We have seen the extent to which the behaviour of long-stay patients is a result of adaptation to their institutionalized environment. Whether the patient loses or retains the behaviours which brought him into hospital originally, as long as he remains in such an environment, he will exhibit socially undesirable behaviour. Because he has *learnt* to adapt to the institutionalized style of life by either acquiring 'new' inappropriate behaviours or losing the appropriate behaviours he once possessed, when he is thrust into a different environment, such as the community, he will continue to display these 'odd' behaviours since they have become part of his repertoire. By learning to adapt to a 'deadening' environment he learns behaviours that will hinder his accommodation in the community. Part of institutionalization of course is the 'binding' of the patient to the institution so he becomes dependent upon it and reluctant to leave it.

Since it appears patients are susceptible to their environment, herein lies the key to their treatment. If an environment can be instrumental in creating such devastating behaviours as social withdrawal, poverty of speech and so on, then if managed appropriately it must also have the potential for creating other behaviours—socially desirable ones. This involves making the patient's living environment the treatment area. For this to be realized, however, the existing rigid and restrictive patterns common to institutional life have to be modified so that a more therapeutic milieu can take place. Only then will treatment succeed. This chapter places accent on modifying the environment in ways both to make life more tolerable for the permanent residents of the institution, and to create an atmosphere where higher level patients can be taught again how to live in the community. Russell Barton suggested that to combat institutionalization, the patient's living environment should encourage:

1. Contact with the outside 'world'
2. Personal possessions and events
3. A homely, permissive ward atmosphere
4. Patient involvement in planning

1. RE-ESTABLISHING CONTACT WITH THE OUTSIDE WORLD

All attempts to re-establish contact start from the ward. The outside world may be a strange place to many patients and anxiety can be unnecessarily caused by suddenly 'dropping them in at the deep end'. We therefore initiate training in the patient's present environment—the ward—and gradually progress to using facilities in other parts of the hospital, until eventually contact with the community can be made.

Doctors, nurses and domestic staff may be the only people whom some patients ever meet who have personal contact with the world outside hospital. Talking with patients about their everyday experiences, such as evening activities, hobbies and family life often creates interest. Spending a few minutes talking to a patient regularly can build up rapport and help him feel someone is interested in him. It is often helpful for each nurse to take responsibility for a small group of patients each day so that relationships can be built up between them, and some time devoted to the teaching or re-acquaintance of various skills such as washing, bed-making and other domestic tasks.

Patients also need to be orientated in time, knowing the day and the season of the year. Where every day is marked by the same routine carried out with unvarying precision (e.g. meals served at exactly the same time each day), and where the nurse prompts the patient into activity every time he is required to perform some behaviour such as getting up, shaving and coming for meals, there is little need for him to know the time, the day or even the month. When, on the other hand, the patient becomes responsible for his own behaviour, where nurses deliberately refrain from prompting the patient, the ability to read the time becomes important in order not to miss a meal or a trip to the cinema by not preparing himself adequately before the event.

Time orientation can be taught to patients. For the most withdrawn it may involve reinstating the skill of reading the clock. For other patients, having a calendar on the ward or being assisted to keep a diary, in which are noted events freshly introduced into the routine such as a trip to town or an especially personal event such as the birthday of a relative, can help them monitor the days.

Visitors who make the occasional visit will be encouraged to come more frequently if they are made to feel welcome. Pens and paper should be made available for patients to write letters to their relatives, initially under nurse supervision, and later when their ability to write has developed to do so unaided. Where such a programme is followed up it can lead to further personal contact. One interesting development after establishing a patient could write a reasonable letter resulted in a number of favourable consequences. This particular patient had a son whom she had not seen for 26 years. After a number of correspondences between the two of them the son began to visit her in hospital. Eventually this led to the patient visiting her son in his home for the day, the nurse first organizing the visit and accompanying the patient. Later the patient was able to spend a weekend with the family taking responsibility for two bus rides each way and planning the visit herself.

The reading of newspapers and watching TV is useful if the patient actively participates, rather than passively takes it in. Special attention paid to local news on radio and television and in the papers can spark off interest and can be used for discussion with patients.

Where sessions are put aside and time made available to teach patients skills which will be required in the community, the use of role play can be valuable. In simulated situations on the ward patients can be taught appropriate behaviours such as shopping, inquiring about a job and even such basic requirements as how to cross the road safely. Many patients resident in hospital for a number of years become unfamiliar with the use of money. Decimal currency is often strange to them, the value of money is totally unrealistic and the ability to budget is non-existent since living has been for the 'here and now'. Plastic toy money may be a way of introducing new currency and again the patient may be helped to value and budget by role playing in simulated situations.

Hospital facilities are often useful to use as a 'stepping stone' to using facilities in the community. After a female patient is taught to keep her hair tidy on the ward, for example, the programme should be extended so she is helped to go to the hairdressers in the hospital, if possible by arranging the times herself. When capable of doing this, the final step is obviously attending a hairdressers in the community. Though a nurse will most probably have to arrange the trip and supervise closely at first, her involvement should gradually decrease and the patient be allowed to plan and organize her own trips.

Patients can be taught how to dance during group sessions and improve their appearance in ward programmes. The natural extension of these skills is to promote them through involvement in hospital socials and dances. This consequently may lead to an evening at a pub or a club in the community. There are a number of ways hospital facilities can be used to aid the patients' treatment in this way. A noticeboard, large and attractive, is useful in letting patients know what events are occurring both on the ward, in the hospital and in the community. Some patients will obviously need to be helped in reading and understanding the notices, but with time and patience this can be achieved.

The final 'test' comes when the patient is taken into the community and attempts to use the facilities. Though some of the skills required will be natural extensions of those acquired on the ward and in the hospital, other skills may have to be specifically taught in the community setting. How to use public conveniences, read a timetable, catch the correct bus, shop sensibly, ask for information at the appropriate places and so on, are some of the necessary skills which require developing.

Planning trips into the community should not be left entirely to the nurse, but patients can participate and involve themselves in a number of ways. Suggesting places to visit, packing up sandwiches if necessary and saving up money for any personal expenses may be the beginning. Later, inquiring about prices, transport and the times of an event may become part of the patient's responsibility. Cafes, picnics, cinemas and sporting events are ways of spending an afternoon in situations outside the hospital, and visits to local places of interest such as factories, art galleries and museums may also be beneficial.

Nurses are involved in each stage of the progression outward to the community, but they should aim to gradually withdraw from the picture so that the patient is eventually able to function independently. Russell Barton stressed the point that 'individual enterprise must be fostered and not smothered by *nurses* doing things the patient might be able to do. The art of the nurse is to judge when to intervene to preserve the patient's dignity and confidence without robbing him of the chance to do things for himself'. For example, if we decide to teach a patient how to use a bus, we must first of all go with him to demonstrate how it should be done. On the next trip, the nurse may allow the patient to buy his ticket and collect the change whilst she stands nearby. When this stage has been established the nurse may decide to stand a few places back in the bus queue and sit a few seats behind the patient on the bus. All the time the nurse 'fades' herself out, always ensuring the patient is capable of functioning adequately at each stage before moving on to the next stage.

2. ENCOURAGE PERSONAL EVENTS AND POSSESSIONS

There may be events and possessions in the patient's environment but these may not necessarily be 'personal'. By personal is meant events which have significance for an individual, and items which are one's own. In looking at a patient's environment, we need first to distinguish between what is personal and what is impersonal and then constantly try and place the accent on the personal.

Choice is normally possible for most patients in a wide range of situations but is rarely exercised. Having a choice in the clothes he wears, his night attire, or rugs and pictures for his own room is preferable to his being given them. It is better still if the patient is able to buy these items with his own money from the hospital shop, or during special visits when local retailers bring a selection of goods and set up stalls in the hospital. The ideal situation, however, is when the patient is able to go into town unaccompanied and purchase items himself. Patients are more likely to care for items they have saved for and purchased themselves, than they are to care for items having no personal significance. There is little point in having something if you cannot use it at your will. Patients need to have their own wardrobe where they can keep their own clothes, shoes, handbags, towels and toilet accessories, preferably having a lock and a key which is in their possession. Some possessions are not so much for use as for display—ornaments, photographs of relatives, birthday cards and holiday postcards—and ideally a locker top or table should be available so these possessions can be displayed.

When patients acquire a 'new' possession, they often need training in how to use the item. The skills involved in using hearing aids, filling cigarette lighters, wearing dentures and using the contents of a wash-bag, may therefore require instruction.

Once a patient possesses an item its effectiveness may depend upon regular maintenance. Therefore patients may need to be taught where to buy a battery for a hearing aid, how to clean their newly acquired dentures and perhaps how to wash their clothes. Minor repairs are constantly cropping up such as the need to sew on buttons, darn a sock or replace a broken shoe lace, and as far as possible facilities should be available for patients to at least attempt such minor repairs themselves. When larger or more delicate repairs need attention, the patient should learn where to go to obtain this—the jewellers if his watch breaks, or the optician if he loses a screw from the hinge of his spectacles, for example.

Patients can also be encouraged to make things for themselves. Cooking his own meal having bought the ingredients himself is a more personal event for the patient than the widely practised, mass catering. The making of a book rack, cushion or scarf at occupational therapy is a more personal experience than buying such items, and the item can be either kept and used by the individual himself or given to a visitor or friend as a present.

Remembering a patient's birthday with cards and giving him a party occurs only once a year. However, there are many events which can be made available throughout the year such as individual shopping expeditions, visits to a pub, cinema or hairdressers. It is not enough simply to arrange for these things to happen, but the patient needs to be involved in the planning and organizing of the event. This may be achieved in a number of ways, such as making items and posters for a sale of work, planning a social on the ward or organizing an inter-ward darts match. Such events become personal and patients begin to look forward to them with increased enthusiasm and remember them with greater pleasure.

Personal involvement again has to be taught to most patients, for they have lived so many years without this participation. For example, one patient had been encouraged for 3 months to save up for a day trip to the seaside, but saved only 9p. On previous trips he had been bought everything, without having to save. On this particular trip he enjoyed the meals provided by the hospital, but was unable to buy the cups of tea, ice cream, rock and shandies enjoyed by his more provident ward-mates. On subsequent trips he saved up to £2, and looked forward to and enjoyed immensely the freedom of spending his own money.

Trips home and regular visits from relatives can be valuable personal events to look forward to. Events supplied by the hospital are better than nothing at all, but events planned, organized and executed by the patients themselves are superior because of the personal involvement.

3. PROVIDE A HOMELY, PERMISSIVE WARD ATMOSPHERE

This does not mean complete licence for patients to do, or not do, as they want, but rather it means a reduction of rules and lessening of regimentation. Rules should be limited in ways that allow patients freedom and preserve their dignity. For example, capable patients should be left to bathe in private rather than have a nurse there to supervise or to do the washing for them. The ostentatious locking of cupboards and doors and restricting patients' privileges such as being put in dressing gowns can also be reduced with a little thought. The aims of the ward should be clearly defined, for if they include rehabilitation with an expectation of leaving hospital, then the ward should not be so comfortable that the motivation to go is reduced. If the aims are not set as high, and where the ward contains patients who have little hope of discharge, then ward life should be made more tolerable for them. It is for such patients that the word 'homely' is used, for they may have to spend the rest of their lives in hospital. Whatever the aims, there is a need to improve the physical environment of long-stay wards to some degree and this can be achieved by paying attention to that which the patients can perceive.

Long-stay wards may have facilities such as cooking utensils, a washing machine, shoe-cleaning equipment, books and a record player, but only too often they are not readily accessible to patients. Usually they are under the control of staff because patients 'don't know how to use them', but effort should be directed at teaching patients how to use and look after such facilities.

Ideally each patient should have the choice of a single room. He should at least be able to create a private space for himself, possibly by having a screen round his bed which he can use at his own discretion. If a patient wants to be apart from other people it helps if they have a chair or stool in their room or by their bed. In this way they are able to enjoy a smoke in peace, away from the pestering of other patients. Where possible a quiet room should be provided, in which patients can entertain visitors or enjoy half an hour reading the paper away from routine noises of the ward.

Flowers, plants, lamps, carpets, tablecloths, wallpaper and pieces of furniture like a bookcase add to the attractiveness of the ward and make it a more pleasant place in which to 'live'. Though mass purchases make for economic 'housekeeping' the monotony of rows of chairs of similar style and colour is not as preferable as the presence of an occasional armchair or a settee around the place. Sometimes wards can be made too 'clinical'—part of a home is the presence of piles of books or magazines, a coat strewn over a chair and a cupboard in a mess.

The activity (or inactivity!) and appearance of patients affects the ward atmosphere. Group activities can be used to alleviate apathy and inactivity by creating interest and focusing on specific behavioural problems. Inappropriate and bedraggled appearance can be improved by clean, modern and well-fitting clothes, and cosmetics for female patients, the provision of which needs to be co-ordinated with training in their appropriate use. The motivation to maintain their appearance can be provided through parties and trips out, whilst mirrors also help to show the patient what he looks like.

Pictures painted by patients can be hung on the walls, and cushions and rugs made at occupational therapy (O.T.) can be used to decorate the ward. Not just any item the patient makes but rather the ones selected by staff and patients as being good, should be displayed, otherwise the feeling 'anything does' may be fostered. Patients can also be encouraged to write out some of the notices which are to be displayed on the ward. Part of some ward tasks can be performed by patients with the co-operation of domestic staff assisting in a supervisory capacity. Sweeping the corridor and mopping the bathroom and toilet floor are two such jobs. Others generally accepted as the responsibility of nurses, such as serving meals and laying the table, can be given the patient. Specific groups, or even formally constituted committees of patients, can be formed to make decisions on ward matters, and to work as teams on ward projects such as decorating for Christmas, or formulating the group activity programme. A ward, for example, may have its own planning committee with patients acting as chairman and secretary.

Of the potential drawbacks in creating ward environments along these lines, there are two of particular concern. Firstly, having stressed the importance of motivating those patients who are potentially capable of living in the community to leave the hospital, we may find that the patient after living in such an environment has come to expect equally good facilities in his 'new' home outside. For example, one patient looking for a flat with a rent she could afford also wanted a refrigerator, washing machine and all the other extras before she would move in. The second drawback, as Russell Barton suggested, is that a ward having good interior decorations and furnishings might present a superficially good impression to visitors, but may persist in creating institutionalized behaviour because other factors not immediately obvious to 'outsiders' are still operating. As we have seen, the understimulating environment can produce institutionalized behaviour such as social withdrawal and poverty of speech. However, moving to the other extreme does not alleviate these. In fact, excessive stimulation can create further undesirable behaviours.

Both excessive physical stimulation, such as noise in the form of constant loud radio, shouting and banging doors; and excessive social stimulation—those situations perceived as 'stressful' by a patient, such as participation in a group discussion or preparing to go down town for the first time—can be distressing to patients. Professor Wing believes 'over' stimulation can lead to an increase in socially embarrassing behaviour such as shouting, pacing, talking to self, delusional or bizarre speech, and aggressive behaviour. Physical stimulation can be reduced with a little thought (e.g. turning the radio down or off for periods of time), but stressful social stimulation is more difficult to tackle. Everyone experiences 'stress' or nervousness in a new situation (such as a new job) but usually adapts to it in a little time and the associated stress is thus reduced. In a therapeutic environment, patients will be confronted by a number of new situations and hence will experience 'stress' quite often. However, if the new situation can be introduced gradually and in small stages, then the level of stress will never be sufficient to cause the patient too much difficulty but will allow him to adapt relatively easily.

4. ENCOURAGE POSITIVE PLANNING BY PATIENTS

Opportunities for patients to plan are often very limited but need to be extended as fully as possible in order to provide opportunities for patients to take responsibility, use their initiative and become motivated to leave hospital. In practice, this means planning events for themselves and for others, planning for employment, for accommodation and financial planning.

Even a simple visit home may involve a great deal of planning; deciding what to take, working out a timetable and estimating the total cost. Other events which may involve quite complex planning are expeditions, visits to the library, a trip to a cricket match, or evening class. Many plans usually worked out by nurses can often be delegated to patients, including interward socials, selecting a team for a darts match, and planning a day trip.

For more able patients, work in the hospital departments should be seen as a step prior to working in the community. Where possible work should be tailored to the patient's needs—his previous occupation and his present state of functioning. He should not be sent to some department and forgotten, as has often occurred. Industrial therapy is only important provided it re-establishes the habit of getting up and to work on time and accepting the kind of discipline which occurs in work situations outside of hospital.

Preparing for work outside involves some knowledge of a wide number of agencies such as good newspapers for job adverts and the location of the Job Centre. Local firms and the Disablement Resettlement Officer (DRO) can be very helpful in finding employment. Initially part-time employment or work at a rehabilitation centre may be advisable, letting the patient lodge at the hospital until full-time employment can be found. Mock interviews where a nurse takes the role of a prospective employer can be very helpful for patients giving them practice in dealing with difficult situations.

When patients have improved sufficiently to leave hospital, the problem of accommodation arises. Relatives might be encouraged to take a patient back into the family, but he may often not have any living nearby or they may be difficult to contact. Often relatives do not want the patient back because he carries the stigma of having lived in a mental hospital, or the relatives have the responsibility of a family or are too old to be able to cope with the patient. In any case it is often not advisable to put patients back with their families, for in doing so the patient may be returned to a situation which may have contributed to his admission in the first place.

If relatives cannot be considered as a source of accommodation, then the search for a place to live is on. The patient has to make a number of decisions during this process:

How much can I afford?

What type of accommodation do I want? A look round a hostel, a half-way house or a group home may help him to make a realistic decision as to where he wants to live. Alternatively he may want to lodge, live in a bedsit or in a flat. The choice should be his, but the advantages and disadvantages of each in relation to the patient's needs, should be spelled out. For example, a dominating person or one who keeps himself to himself may not be suited to a group home, where the individuals have to learn to live together as a group.

Where do I want to live? If he chooses a place too near the hospital, there is a danger that the links will never be broken. He may be resident 'outside' but for all intents and purposes still 'live' in the hospital by attending social events and perhaps even meals inside the institution. Where the accommodation is in an area away from the hospital, voluntary bodies may be only too willing to make friends with the patient, show him around the area and help him to find shops, launderettes and so on.

Where do I look for vacancies? Patients may be taught to look through the local newspapers or other local publications, to glance at the small advertisements in shop windows or go to an estate agent. An enquiry about accommodation may involve making a telephone call or writing, both of which the patient should have been taught. Help may be given him when he goes to visit the property, so he can be sure of making the correct decision upon whether or not to accept the vacancy.

When he moves from the hospital, links should be maintained to some extent through visits from community nurses and maybe returning to work in the Day Hospital. However the patient should be encouraged to live his own life, away from the hospital, for example, by finding a local GP and developing interests in community organizations.

Long-stay patients frequently operate on day-to-day budget, so they need to understand why and how to save. Opening and using a bank account or Post Office savings account, budgeting and choosing from a range of goods which look roughly the same but vary in cost and usefulness are all necessary skills the patient needs on discharge.

If we look closely at the patient's environment, and become aware of the processes operating in it, we can reduce those operating in an anti-therapeutic manner, and reverse them so that progress occurs in place of decline.

Chapter 6

NURSE–PATIENT INTERACTION

The importance of nurses in the treatment of patients has been recognized for almost as long as there have been psychiatric institutions. One record of 1861 stated, 'Nothing in connection with the treatment of the insane has a more direct and immediate effect, for good or ill, upon their condition and comfort, than the fact of their being under the charge of good or bad attendants'. What constitutes the 'good' nurse of today is her ability to realize and utilize the enormous therapeutic potential she has.

We have stressed the importance of modifying the patients' environment in combating institutionalization, but the most significant events in the patients' environment are the activities of other people. Nurses, being the only group of staff who are with patients most of the day, therefore form a significant proportion of the environment and are thus in an ideal position to interact with patients in a therapeutic way. Nurses are also very often the only contact patients have with the outside world, and therefore they act as both a 'model' or example and informant of the skills society expects. The nurse can thus become the key person in a patient's treatment, her attitudes and type of interaction being of fundamental importance in modifying the behaviour of long-stay patients.

NATURE OF SOCIAL INTERACTION

Social interaction occurs when two people meet and acknowledge each other. Joan may meet Doris on the street. They may meet as strangers, as business companions, as neighbours, as friends or even meet on unfriendly terms, and this relationship will obviously affect how interaction between the two of them will proceed. During any interaction, however, no matter of what type it is, a tremendous amount of information is conveyed from one to the other. This is usually at three levels:

1. The content, or the intentions of what is meant to be said.
2. The expression, or the inflection—how the information is

conveyed. The mood of a person, for example, is apparent in the way he talks—faster when anxious, slower when depressed and louder when angry. In addition the way different words are emphasized or stressed conveys the function of a statement. Inflection therefore enables the recipient of a message to distinguish whether a statement is a question or a command. Written statements, in contrast, contain no inflection and may therefore be taken to mean a number of different things—one humorous example is found on British Rail WCs: 'Gentlemen lift the seat'. Is this a command, a definition or a loyal toast?

3. The non-verbal information, communicated by way of gestures, postures and facial expressions. The importance of such information is often overlooked, although intuitively people often respond very sensitively to non-verbal information. Eye contact is a common way of showing interest, hand movements emphasize points and postures convey mood—for example, people tend to sit upright when tense and slouch when relaxed.

In an interaction, the way Doris behaves in response to what Joan says will determine how the interaction proceeds. Doris's reaction, if verbal, will contain information at the three levels of content, inflection and non-verbal information, but even if she makes no verbal response, she will all the time be communicating non-verbally with Joan. If Doris wants Joan to carry on speaking, she may attend to what is being said, nod her head in agreement and probably interject with a 'Hum' or 'Yes' occasionally. However, when Doris wants to add anything or raise a special issue she has to notify Joan of her intentions by attracting Joan's attention through hand gestures and butting in verbally whenever there is a pause. If either of them want to end a particular line of conversation, this may effectively be achieved by looking uninterested or by changing the subject of discussion.

Between people with a similar cultural background there usually exist unspoken but commonly accepted rules of interaction. Conversations can therefore be modified, extended or closed depending upon the participants' reactions to one another's utterances. Interactions between two people are very complicated, and as they involve both verbal and non-verbal elements, ample opportunity exists for misinterpretation. For example, an over-enthusiastic non-verbal reaction by one person, such as moving closer to the other, may be interpreted by the other as a threatening gesture. When the two people are recent acquaintances each has to learn what is acceptable to the other to reduce the chance of misinterpretation.

NURSE–PATIENT INTERACTION

In the study of institutionalization we saw that where nurses interact with patients it is frequently in an unsystematic and antitherapeutic way, though the nurse usually has the concern of the patient at heart. Her behaviour is often the result of the training she has been subjected to, which, like the doctors', is structured around the medical model. This perpetuates the nurse in the role of medical aide, offering little in the way of developing her therapeutic potential. We aim now to look a little deeper into some of the ways nurses traditionally feel about and interact with patients, and how such encounters can be structured in a more therapeutic way.

We will look at four aspects:
1. The nurses' attitude
2. Attending to undesirable behaviour
3. Lack of interaction
4. Stereotyped interaction

1. THE NURSES' ATTITUDE

The way we think and feel about something obviously affects the way we behave. If, for example, our attitude towards chronic schizophrenic patients is that they have a hopeless prognosis, then this will inevitably be communicated to the patient in various ways, and we would hardly be motivated to set about treating his problems.

Our attitudes are formed and affected by our knowledge and experience. Nurses on long-stay wards work in environments which are conducive to the development of attitudes which are not always beneficial for the patient. Therefore, in order to help chronic patients, feelings towards them may need modifying. The most important attitudes to promote are:

(a) Long-stay patients can be treated
(b) Nurses can treat
(c) Empathy—considering the patient's point of view
(d) Patients are people
(e) Patients are individuals
(f) Assets are more important than defects

(a) *Long-stay patients can be treated.* Hospitals exist to treat, yet often all a patient may receive apart from a few tranquillizers is three meals a day, a bed to sleep in, adequate clothing and warmth. Custodial care leaves untreated the behavioural problems of the patient, which are, in part at least, the reason why he is still in hospital. Years of unfruitful results with long-stay patients often leave the nurse with a pessimistic 'Well what can you do, we've tried everything' attitude. However, there is hope for long-stay patients. The systematic approach of rehabilitation units throughout the country has demonstrated that patients can be taught to live in the community again. Even the most withdrawn patient is capable of improving to some degree through the application of behavioural techniques which have, for example, reduced the number of incidents of incontinence and aggression. Only when the nursing staff see that results can be obtained with such techniques can they be expected to be sympathetic towards the treatment, but once their enthusiasm is kindled, the chronic patient's future can look bright.

(b) *Nurses can treat*. Nurses, by tradition, often think of treatment as something carried out or initiated by the doctor, but in the treatment of long-stay patients, the nurse is as important, if not *more* important than the doctor. Having the greatest degree of contact with patients, the nurse has a greater potential for influencing behaviour, and should therefore become the major agent of treatment, being able to initiate treatment on her own behalf.

(c) *Empathy*. By trying to put ourselves in the patient's position, we can greatly increase our understanding of his problems. Rather than accepting the patient's problems as an inevitable part of his personality we should become more acutely aware of the effects of institutionalization, the particular problems which face a patient and of the enormous influence we ourselves, as nurses, have on the patient's behaviour. We are then able to start questioning our own behaviour and begin to judge what the consequences of our behaviour might be before acting. 'How is this going to affect the patient?' or 'What are the consequences of doing this?' may be questions worth considering before interacting with a patient in a particular traditional way. We may therefore become aware of the need to tolerate slower or poorer performance, to reduce prompting and allow patients to make more decisions on their own.

(d) *Patients are people*. Often patients are thought of as 'mad', 'bad' or 'childish', and even if it is not openly stated, the tone of voice and choice of words used by staff may clearly show they think of patients in a condescending sub-adult way. Patients may be shouted at, reprimanded for minor ward infringements, talked about in their presence and, if they are a 'textbook case', may be singled out and shown to visitors.

Patients ought to be treated as any other person should be treated: given time, listened to and asked their opinion on matters concerning their welfare. One useful technique for doing this is frequently to ask ourself, 'Would I act like that with someone outside?', and if the answer is positive then at least the way is opened for the patient to start behaving normally. If we start to expect 'normal' things from patients, we may start finding they behave accordingly. People usually behave in ways expected of them, and so if we think of patients as mad or childish how can we expect them to behave normally?

Behaviour can be changed through expectations. Rosenthal and Jacobson, in an interesting study carried out in a school situation, told class teachers that on the basis of a carefully collected set of test results, some of the children were expected to improve noticeably, while others would not. At the end of the year the children selected as likely to improve did so, while the others did not. However, both groups of children were initially the same, chosen at random from the total class. The difference between the two groups was only in the teachers' expectations about the children.

The same effect was noted with insulin coma therapy, patients improving because they and the staff expected they would, not because of a demonstrable treatment effect due to insulin alone. When we expect something to happen, we behave in ways to bring this about, perhaps through giving patients more attention, interacting differently with them, or organizing their day in different ways.

(e) *Patients are individuals.* A patient will often be grouped and categorized in various ways, so that he is not seen as an individual in his own right, but is labelled in terms of those behaviours which represent the group. For example, a patient may be labelled a schizophrenic, low grade or high grade (depending upon the level of job he is able to perform), an absconder or an incontinent patient, rather than being seen as an individual person with a number of unique problems.

Individual activities and choice require fostering and nurses should not be afraid to take a personal interest in patients. Individualizing our approach can only be established by getting to know each patient well—something of his likes, his dislikes, his background and hopes—and in achieving this, there is no substitute for spending time constructively with a patient. Once we get to know a patient, interaction becomes more natural and we are able to:

(i)   Have some idea of how he is likely to react to us, and how he will interpret our behaviour. Some patients respond to a lot of attention from nurses, whilst others respond better if left more on their own.

(ii) Know what level of vocabulary to use. Some patients may not understand words we commonly use with our colleagues and friends.

(iii) Know how fast or loud to speak. Some patients become confused if people speak too fast, or if they do not pronounce words clearly.

(iv) Know how much he understands and can retain. It is possible for us to ask a patient to do something, and for him to say 'Yes' when asked if he has understood, but five minutes later for him to have obviously forgotten what was said. We may have to give information in parts so it can be 'taken in'. On the other hand, it is often easy to underestimate what a patient can understand. One very withdrawn patient, for example, when given a series of four instructions on how to change her clothes, wash her dress, comb her hair and wash her face went away and performed all the tasks without any further prompting, much to everybody's surprise.

(*f*) *Assets are more important than defects.* All too often the major emphasis is on controlling and punishing what patients do wrong. Minor infringements are highlighted and the parts of a task the patient does inadequately are emphasized, probably because it is inefficient and thus affects the smooth running of the routine. However, environments become therapeutic when the good aspects of a patient's performance are sought and highlighted. For example, telling a patient he has had four dry beds a week rather than telling him he has had three wet ones, is a positive approach and more likely to succeed. Concentrating upon the good aspects and building these up communicates enthusiasm to the patient, whereas concentrating upon the worse aspects creates punitive situations.

2. ATTENDING TO UNDESIRABLE BEHAVIOUR

Nurses and patients interact in many ways, but they are not always therapeutic. As we have seen, inappropriate behaviour is frequently reinforced by nursing staff and adaptive behaviour tends to be ignored. One study reported that over 90% of patients' adaptive behaviour failed to be recognized by staff which suggests the majority of nurses' attention was directed towards undesirable behaviour, probably because smashing windows, lying on the floor and attempts at suicide, for example, disrupt the smooth and efficient running of the daily routine. The patient who causes no trouble, but sits in the same chair all day, rarely speaking, and has to be prompted to come for his meals, is seen to be the 'good' patient, for by passively complying with the routine he causes the nurse no extra effort. On the other hand, the more active and independent patient makes surveillance more difficult and so is not encouraged to behave in this more appropriate way. Additionally, a patient's behaviour may capture attention because of its odd or unusual nature. Gelfand and his colleagues found nurses paid attention to a fair proportion of the odd and unusual speech of their patients, while not paying a great deal more attention to their normal appropriate speech.

The inappropriate or unusual aspects of a behaviour stand out against the normal or expected behaviour, and therefore often come in for a fair amount of attention. The poorer aspects of a patient's work, the deficits in his appearance or the inappropriateness of his table manners are therefore more easily noticed and focused on by nurses at the expense of the more frequent but less apparent assets in the patient's behaviour. This in turn leads to nurses using 'negative' rather than positive words such as 'can't', 'shouldn't', 'wouldn't', 'never', and 'don't'. When such words are used in sentences directed at patients, we frequently hear comments like '*Dont't* eat with your knife' or 'Why *haven't* you brushed your hair?' thus drawing attention again to the undesirable behaviour.

These examples serve to illustrate how undesirable behaviour may be increased and maintained usually quite unwittingly, through nurse–patient interaction. Treatment involves an entirely different approach to patients' behaviour—often the reverse of what commonly occurs. It requires the structuring of nurse–patient interaction in ways which increase desirable behaviour and decrease undesirable behaviour. This can be achieved through behaviour modification.

The attractiveness of *behaviour modification* as a treatment method lies in its simplicity—it is as simple as A, B, C for it is based on:

Antecedents—the situation which causes the behaviour to occur.
Behaviour—the occurrence of the behaviour itself.
Consequences—the consequences of a behaviour, or what happens after a behaviour has been performed.

All behaviour has antecedents and consequences. For example, a headache (antecedent) might cause us to take some medication (behaviour) which could relieve the pain (consequence); or the quest for further knowledge (antecedent) might prompt us to ask a question (behaviour) which is answered by the tutor (consequence).

The consequence of a behaviour affects the frequency of the occurrence of that behaviour. Take, for example, the behaviour of joke telling. Should we tell a joke at work and our colleagues laugh, then we might tell the joke again in the company of different people. The behaviour of joke telling has been increased. If, however, the audience remain silent we would be unlikely to tell the joke again. The good consequence (e.g. laughter at our joke) is called a *positive reinforcer* and the behaviour which has increased has been *reinforced* (or strengthened).

A positive reinforcer is any stimulus which increases the probability of a response. A weekly wage positively reinforces attendance at a job since payment is contingent upon time spent at work. Similarly we see that if nurses' attention is a reinforcer for a patient, and he can obtain this attention through bizarre speech or lying on the floor, then these undesirable behaviours will increase because they are reinforced.

Behaviour can also be increased by *negative reinforcers*—that is where behaviour is strengthened by the escape or avoidance of a particular consequence. For example, a housewife may persist in cooking nice meals to avoid her husband's complaints. By obeying traffic signals we are being negatively reinforced because by doing so we avoid legal punishment (an unpleasant stimulus). One therapist introduced a loud unpleasant noise (negative reinforcer) through a hidden loud-speaker whenever a therapy group of schizophrenic patients fell silent for more than one minute. As soon as a patient broke the silence, the noise was turned off and within a few sessions the group was converted from a near silent one to a lively talkative group.

Often positive and negative reinforcement operate together to maintain a behaviour. For example, a heavy drinker may persist with this behaviour because when he drinks it helps him feel relaxed and at peace with the world (he is positively reinforced), and he escapes from those things which are worrying him (negatively reinforced).

Positive reinforcers are frequently called 'rewards' because they are experienced as pleasant, but it is important that a reinforcer is not defined by its intrinsic properties or subjective feelings but rather by the effect it has on a behaviour. A stimulus only becomes a reinforcer when it actually results in an increase in the frequency of a behaviour.

This may be illustrated with the teetotaller who spent an hour cleaning up a hall after a concert. The organizer wanting to reward him for his help gave him a bottle of whisky, which, though seen as a reward by the organizer, was not a reinforcer for it would not prompt the teetotaller to help again. Rewards are subjective, whereas reinforcers are objective. Those events or stimuli which increase the behaviour they are contingent upon are positive reinforcers, whereas those events that increase behaviour which avoids or escapes the stimulus are negative reinforcers.

The art of treatment is to arrange contingencies between behaviour and its consequences so that desirable behaviour is followed by pleasant consequences and undesirable behaviour receives no such reinforcement. Nurses may be in the habit of using such contingencies already, so that certain privileges may be contingent upon acceptable ward behaviour. However, as Schaefer and Martin have pointed out, the behaviour therapist insists that complete consistency is maintained in manipulating such contingencies and that many more immediate consequences are arranged. They say 'Behaviour therapy involves the complete structuring of a patient's environment and is made as all-encompassing as possible. . . almost all necessities as well as luxuries of daily life are made contingent upon some behaviour'.

The nurse–patient encounter is an ideal situation in which to practise reinforcement, since the nurse herself is a potential source of social reinforcers. Interactions should be structured so that there is an aim for each patient and a specified means to achieve this aim, since it will differ for each individual with respect to his particular problem. In a ward situation, the most appropriate procedures the nurse can use in her approach are the social ones—attention, praise and extinction—which she can structure in ways to treat a patient's problems.

Attention

Being social creatures we like the company of other people. During social encounters we are continually reinforcing each other by the attention we give and receive. Similarly the attention nurses give patients reinforces their behaviour. If given for undesirable behaviour rather than appropriate behaviour, a nurse could unwittingly cause the patient's state to deteriorate. Treatment should involve giving attention contingent upon appropriate acts and ignoring inappropriate behaviour, an approach which is not limited to specified types of behaviour or to a specific type of patient. Ways of giving attention include:

Sitting next to a patient.
Listening to him.
Looking at him (especially eye contact).
Conversing with him.
Showing interest in what he is doing.

Using words or doing things in a way which draws out an emotional response from a patient will act as a reinforcer. Using words such as fun, holiday, laughter, party, the patient's home town and so on in sentences when in conversation may help an interaction become even more reinforcing for the patient.

Giving attention to appropriate behaviour is a useful technique for increasing behaviour, but it is not a reinforcer for all patients. In fact some patients will learn behaviours in order to avoid any contact with other people. For these patients other reinforcers need to be found.

Praise

Praising behaviour follows the same principles as paying attention to behaviour—it increases or maintains the frequency of a behaviour it follows. If a patient is praised for being prompt at a meal he may be encouraged to be prompt more often. Praise includes any way of communicating to the patient he has done well and involves both non-verbal (smiles, head nods or a pat on the back) and verbal communications. Effective verbal praise appears to differ between individuals, so that being told 'correct' might reinforce a scientist, while a working factory-hand might respond better to 'good'. The nurse who starts to praise patients makes available new sources of reinforcement for the individual patient, who may then start to orientate himself to attend the new social aspects of his environment.

It may often appear as if there is nothing to reinforce in a patient's performance, but we should always strive to find positive aspects in his behaviour. Thus if a patient sweeps the corridor with the brush upside down, he has at least taken the brush from the cupboard. This would be where we start to reinforce him with a comment like, 'Well done, I see you've got the brush out ready to start'. From this point we are in a position to build up his behaviour. Such an approach avoids the patient's defects and concentrates upon his virtues. This also leads to the use of positive words rather than negative words and thus directs the patient's attention to the good aspects of his behaviour.

Applying reinforcers. The effectiveness of any reinforcer depends upon how it is given to the patient. The best results occur where nurses:

(i) Reinforce *contingent on appropriate behaviour* NOT inappropriate behaviour. A situation may occur where the behaviour we want to reinforce is accompanied by some inappropriate behaviour which we want to extinguish. For example, a patient sweeping the corridor (desirable behaviour) may be swearing (undesirable behaviour) at the same time. To praise the patient here would be to reinforce both his sweeping and his swearing. To avoid accidentally reinforcing such inappropriate behaviour we have to arrange the situation so that he will be reinforced only when he is sweeping *and not* swearing.

(ii) Reinforce *consistently*. Everyone involved in the patient's treatment must be aware of the approach being used and be able to carry it out correctly. One nurse not sympathetic towards the method of treatment can destroy any amount of work put in by all the other nurses.

(iii) Reinforce *immediately* the desired behaviour occurs, otherwise the association between a particular behaviour and the subsequent reinforcement may not be clear to the patient. The longer the time gap between behaviour and reinforcement, the less effective it will be.

(iv) Reinforce *genuinely*. Nurses often say it is difficult to praise patients—that it seems 'false' giving so much. With increased knowledge of the patients, however, the same nurses say it no longer feels false, but that they want to praise patients because they have done well. Praise should be expressed in a manner which is natural to the nurse and acceptable to the patient. If not, the patient might perceive and interpret it as a punishment, because non-verbal cues may be inconsistent with what is said. For example, 'Well done' said reluctantly or without enthusiasm lacks the appropriate expression and has associated non-verbal elements such as the lack of a smile, which can be picked up by patients.

(v) *Emphasize* praise. Make it quite clear to the patient he has done well. Some patients may fail to respond to non-verbal cues because they avoid eye contact and so they have to be told they have done well.

(vi) Use a *flexible* approach. Continued use of the same phrase such as 'Well done, Johnny' following every bit of desirable behaviour becomes monotonous and loses some of its effectiveness as a reinforcer. Praise should be varied, using phrases such as 'Good', 'That's terrific', 'Smashing', 'You've done very well this time', and sometimes a smile or a nod will do just as well.

(vii) *Give information feedback.* When we praise someone, we usually express why we are making such a gesture. For example, statements like, 'Good, I'm glad you were able to come this time' or 'It's good to see you looking so well' give feedback or informational feedback to the person. We have fed back, as it were, to the original person the reasons for our behaviour. Similarly when we praise patients, it is often wise to tell them why we praise them, so that they can associate our reaction with what they themselves have just done. Without feedback the patient may be rather hazy as to what is being praised. He may not, for example, perceive it as being for talking to another patient, but possibly for wearing a pink tie or smoking a cigarette-end which he may have been doing during the time when he was being reinforced.

Extinction

We have considered how desirable behaviour can be increased by using contingent reinforcement, but how do we treat inappropriate behaviour when it appears in the patient's behavioural repertoire? We should aim to decrease this, and one method by which this can be achieved is *extinction.* A behaviour which is no longer followed by positive reinforcers will decrease in frequency so that in the ward setting when undesirable behaviour occurs it should receive no reinforcement whatsoever. The attention patients obtained previously from nurses through bizarre talk, odd postures, messy table manners and so on, which probably reinforced the patient's behaviour, should be withheld. Ways of doing this include:

Moving away from the person concerned.

Showing no interest in their behaviour, by looking away or shifting attention to other things on the ward.

Starting to do something different which is unrelated to the patient such as counting loose change, looking bored or acting busy.

Extinction ensures inappropriate behaviour is not reinforced, although of course an element of mild punishment may be involved. As the patient's odd beliefs are not confirmed and his outburst of shouting receives no reinforcement, so he begins to look for other ways of behaving to gain attention. For this reason it is not enough simply to ignore the patient's inappropriate behaviour, for he is then deprived of a certain amount of social reinforcement. If he is accustomed to receiving attention he may begin to exhibit other behaviours, likely to be inappropriate ones, to recapture the involvement of the staff. The art is to reinforce behaviour which is both *adaptive* and *incompatible* with his inappropriate behaviour. This was demonstrated by Ayllon and Haughton in a now famous study of 'Kathy', a patient whose speech contained delusional ideas 50% of the time. Nurses were asked to pay attention to normal speech and ignore speech with a delusional content whenever they interacted with Kathy; normal speech being incompatible and more adaptive than delusional speech. Her bizarre speech consequently dropped to 15% of the total speech, and though delusional speech was not removed altogether, it demonstrated that the way a nurse reacts to a patient's behaviour can substantially influence the expression of delusional ideas.

There are three distinct disadvantages in using extinction to reduce behaviour. First, extinction produces only a gradual decrease in behaviour. A patient may therefore have 20 or 30 aggressive outbursts before the behaviour finally extinguishes. An initial effect of extinction is to make the undesirable behaviour occur more frequently. The patient in a sense exaggerates or worsens his behaviour in order to capture the attention he once was used to receiving for engaging in the behaviour. Secondly, during extinction we may be unable to control all the reinforcements the patient receives for performing a certain behaviour so should we decide to ignore a patient's bizarre speech he may not receive attention from nurses, but he might discover other people (patients, domestic staff, etc.) who are willing to listen to him and thus reinforce this undesirable speech. Finally, some behaviours are so destructive we could not afford to let them occur 20 or 30 times. The slashing of wrists or head banging are two examples where extinction would not be an appropriate method to use.

3. LACK OF INTERACTION

Miss A. Altschul's research into nurse–patient interaction has unearthed some interesting findings, and though most of it has been conducted on acute wards, the results and implications are of relevance to those working on long-stay wards. She defined an interaction as an event where a nurse and a patient talked with each other for 5 minutes or over and found:

(a) some 40% of patients did not interact with staff; (b) some staff members failed to interact with patients; (c) the longer a patient stayed in hospital the less likely he was to interact; and (d) the more a nurse progressed up the hierarchical ladder, the less she entered into interaction.

The first three results suggest a general poverty of interaction between nurses and patients. There are many reasons why such a lack of interaction should occur which include:

(i) The patient's difficulty in interacting. For interaction to proceed smoothly between two people, without there being lengthy silences a great deal of social skill is required. It has been reported that schizophrenic patients have difficulty in this skill, plus the fact that their environment is often not conducive to creating events interesting enough to talk about.

(ii) The social structure of a mental hospital makes a truly therapeutic relationship between staff and patients very difficult because of the identification of the former with arbitrary authority.

(iii) Nurses are often told not to get involved or have feelings for patients, otherwise the nurse's own feelings might come to interfere with the carrying out of her duties; but there can be no meaningful human relationship into which feelings do not enter.

(iv) Talking to patients as an activity in itself, apart from seeking and supplying information relevant to the patients' stay in hospital or persuading them to accept some prescribed treatment, is given low priority. It is often a residual activity to be considered if no other jobs on the ward can be found, as illustrated in the not uncommon instruction to nurses 'There's nothing else to do so you might as well talk to the patients'.

Talking with patients should be given a higher priority by nurses than the more routine aspects of basic nursing like bed-making and cleaning. Nurses are well trained in technical aspects of nursing and in formal etiquette, but little or no help has been given in the past to the understanding and management of human relationships. Yet this is essential for the modern nurse. Relationships can be formed only through interaction, but the time spent talking to patients should be spent constructively—social enrichment of the environment is not enough. For interactions to become therapeutic they should be structured so that contingencies are made on the performance of good behaviour. It is the quality of an interaction which is important therapeutically, not the quantity.

Settings need to be provided where people can come together so that interaction between nurse–patient and patient–patient occurs. This can be achieved in a variety of group activities and in situations on the ward such as meal times. Through the formation of relationships nurses find they take more interest in the patients' progress, hobbies, etc., and can act more naturally with patients, in a warm and relaxed manner.

4. STEREOTYPED INTERACTION

Three common yet antitherapeutic types of interaction are often found on long-stay wards:

(a) The paradoxical question—when the patient is asked something such as has he got his socks on and then the nurse proceeds to check, making the patient's response redundant.

(b) Prompting—a lot of interaction between nurses and patients follows a pattern where the nurse instructs the patient to carry out some behaviour (e.g. 'Sit there', 'Come for your tea', 'Put your red dress on', 'Go and fetch your knitting'). Such interaction is antitherapeutic, leaving the patient little room to respond verbally, or to make a decision on his own since the nurse takes the initiative from him.

(c) 'If you do—then' type of interaction. This is a type of prompting which informs the patient that should he perform a certain behaviour he will be rewarded. However, when the patient fails to respond appropriately on a few occasions, it is not uncommon for the prompt to turn to a 'If you don't—then' threat. Examples of this type of interaction are 'If you don't come for your meal right away you'll miss it' or 'If you dirty that dress, you won't get another clean one today'.

These types of interaction can be reduced by teaching the patient to use his initiative and start controlling his own behaviour rather than being dependent on the nurse. Teaching patients to 'think' again can be achieved by:

(a) Letting the patient experience the consequences of his own behaviour. Rather than prompting him to come for his meals, to the ward shop, to have a wash and so on, he should be allowed to discover that what he does, or does not do, has consequences for him. The patient who fails to save up to go to the cinema, or one who throws his dinner purposefully on the floor should also realize the consequences of his behaviour, i.e. he misses the trip out, or loses his meal respectively. It is important again to reinforce any signs of initiative shown by the patient such as having a wash on his own, or asking to clean his own shoes.

(b) Set the patient problems—not unsolvable ones, but small problems which require a solution, when and where he is motivated to do so. Not setting him a knife and fork at the meal table, for example, might prompt him to find solutions to resolve his problem. If his response is appropriate, such as fetching the utensils from the kitchen, or asking a nurse where they are, then he should be reinforced.

(c) Give the patient choice. Presenting the patient with alternatives from which he has to choose requires him to start thinking. What colour dress does she want? Does he want to spend his money at the pub or to save for a transistor radio? What does he want for dinner? These are examples of the many chances there are of giving patients choice and setting them thinking. When the patient has decided, he will usually be naturally reinforced through the privilege he has chosen to enjoy.

(d) Give the patient responsibility. Giving patients small jobs on the wards such as looking after the plants or serving meals, and involving them both in personal planning and planning for a group of patients, produce situations which require the patient to start thinking and organizing.

(e) Fade the prompts given to patients. This involves the gradual removal of the nurse's assistance so the patient develops the ability to perform a behaviour without supervision. For example, if a patient finishes the job of sweeping a corridor and we want him to put the brush away, the stages might be:

    (i)   Verbal prompt (directed) e.g. 'Put the brush in the cupboard now you've finished.'

   (ii)   Verbal prompt (undirected) e.g. 'Now where should the brush go?'

  (iii)   Non-verbal prompt, e.g. glance at cupboard.

  (iv)   No prompt.

By successively using such stages, the amount of information given to the patient is gradually being reduced, and consequently the patient has to think more and more for himself. Verbal prompts can either be *directed* or *undirected*. Direct prompts specify the action desired of the patient. 'Put your coat on' and 'Straighten your tie' are two examples of such prompts, which are extremely common in hospital situations. The patient can perform the skill but relies on the nurse to initiate it, and because the prompt specifies the action desired it leaves little for the patient to think about. Continued use of such prompting deprives the patient of any chance to use his initiative and so we should always attempt to reduce directed prompts. Undirected prompts also initiate action, but do not specify what is desired of the patient—only that something is expected of him. 'What have you forgotten?' and 'Where should you be at this time?' are examples of such prompts, leaving the patient with a problem requiring the use of his initiative in order to solve it. Non-verbal prompts or cues are common experiences for everyone, producing and responding to them frequently in our everyday existence. Alarm clocks, looking at our watch to hint that we want to end a conversation or banging the door when angry are all prompts or cues. The use of hand gestures and eye contact as prompts for patients is useful for they provide less information still for the patient to work on, requiring him to use his initiative even further.

APPLICATION TO SPECIFIC PROBLEMS

The basic principle of behaviour modification—that of positively reinforcing appropriate behaviour and extinguishing undesirable behaviour—is appropriate for the treatment of most problems of long-stay patients, but the way this principle is applied differs in almost every case. This becomes apparent if we compare the treatment of three examples of speech disorder. These examples give a general idea of how treatment of each can be approached, but it must be remembered that the specific details of treatment for each patient will differ for each individual.

Poverty of speech (e.g. monosyllabic speech)
The goal should not be to make patients into public speakers, but to develop their repertoire in ways which will enable them to function

adequately in society so that, for example, they become capable of asking for items at the shop. A start is to structure situations on the ward whereby patients have to ask for what they want at the food trolley, or ask for a light for their cigarette rather than being given one automatically when a gesture is made.

Concentrating on topics the patient is interested in, be it farming, music or whatever, and asking open questions rather than closed questions are more likely to produce lengthy responses. Closed questions are those where the patient can respond with 'Yes', or 'No' and therefore do not extend the patient's speech. 'Do you like this ward?' or 'Is this your own coat?' are examples of closed questions. Open questions on the other hand cannot be answered so simply and therefore require more from the patient. Such questions are 'Where did you used to work?' and 'What did you have for dinner?'

Structured situations like role play, drama groups or quizzes may provide patients with the chance to read aloud written texts or initiate speech. Reinforcement should follow any attempt by the patient to initiate speech and on those occasions where he makes an effort to respond to a question appropriately.

Delusional speech

Wherever possible 'bizarre' speech should be first checked for elements of authenticity, for its content may well be based on truth. For example, one patient who had delusions of grandeur stated that he had once boxed a well-known fighter. This was taken to be more evidence in support of his diagnosis, until he produced a photograph to support his claim.

As Schaefer and Martin have stressed, it is the verbalization of the delusion which marks the patient—a patient who held odd beliefs but did not express them would be considered normal by the people of our society. Treatment should therefore concentrate on reducing the verbal expression of the delusional ideas. Delusions cannot be altered by reasoning or argument, a fact recognized as long ago as 1899 when a nursing textbook stated the effect would only be to concentrate attention on the false beliefs and cause the delusion to become more fixed. The authors suggested that the best way was 'to avoid the subject as much as possible'.

This is still the best remedy, with the addition of reinforcing sensible and rational speech. Speech containing delusional ideas should receive no reinforcement, but giving feedback (e.g. 'I'm sorry, but that doesn't make sense to me') may help, along with directing the conversation away from topics the patient has delusional ideas about. There are schools of thought which believe that the verbal expression of a delusion maintains it, so that depriving the patient of the chance to express it might cause the delusional idea to slowly die away.

Thought disorder

As indicated in Chapter 1, there are many types of thought disorder, and as they manifest themselves in the patient's speech, the aim of treatment is to modify inappropriate speech. The more incoherent a patient's speech, the more interested the audience often seems to be, and so incoherent speech tends to be reinforced.

In the ward setting, the nurse can be instrumental in changing the patient's speech by attending to normal rational speech when it occurs and ignoring inappropriate speech. Schaefer and Martin found that giving patients informational feedback when their speech was inappropriate (e.g. 'That's crazy talk, and I'm not listening to crazy talk') was better than simply walking away, because it gave the nurse a self-produced control stimulus to change her behaviour from listening to non-listening. In addition, a verbal level is attached to the patient's behaviour which may serve to help the patient learn to discriminate between 'crazy' and 'not crazy' talk.

In contrast, it is of no advantage and perhaps detrimental to accompany reasonable talk with statements like, 'That's good reasonable talking', as this sounds condescending and might have an aversive effect. The attention of the listener, his agreements, disagreements and answers are the reinforcers which sustain reasonable talk for all human beings.

One method of helping patients who wander off the point to speak more reasonably is to ask concrete rather than abstract questions and personal rather than impersonal questions. For example, asking a patient to describe happiness (abstract) or the workings of parliament (impersonal) are more likely to produce rambling incoherent speech than are questions about money (concrete) or his former job (personal).

Chapter 7

ETHICAL CONSIDERATIONS

Ethics is defined in the dictionary as 'a set of high moral standards, adopted by an individual person and by which that person endeavours to conduct his life'—as a 'science of morals'; as the 'study of the principles of humanity'; and as 'rules of conduct'.

As carers for sick, infirm and socially inadequate people we, as nurses, need to be sympathetic as well as practical people. The very nature of our work demands not only that we be efficient managers and technicians, but also that we develop an awareness of sensitivity to our patients as people, rather than as recipients of treatment and care. The establishment of a good relationship between nurse and patient is considered, like the traditional 'bedside' manner of the doctor, to ease the patient's anxiety, gain his confidence and involvement in treatment, and provide comfort for him in periods of extreme distress. Our particular relationships and behaviour toward each patient need to be understood and guidelines to such understanding lie in the subject of *ethics*. However, the above sample of dictionary definitions is more likely to provoke further questions than lead to an immediate and profound understanding of the meaning of ethics in practical terms.

If we accept the necessity for understanding the meaning of ethics, we need to translate the abstract quality of these dictionary definitions into forms which are relevant to our experience of daily life and to consider their practical application to our work of nursing. While appreciating that no single brief definition of ethics can do justice to its total meaning, we hope the following definition will serve as a guide to the fundamental aspect of this subject. Our broadly based but simple definition of ethics is: 'Acting towards another person in a considerate manner which preserves that person's dignity and respects his or her right to be treated as an individual human being.'

This definition reflects the philosophy of all social relationships between members of a civilized community and assumes this is the basic aim underlying our relationship with patients. That these aims are identical is no mere coincidence, but the assumption that we *do* treat patients in the same manner as we act towards other people may be rudely shaken when we examine certain ethical aspects of our relationships with 'long-stay' patients.

THE PRACTICAL APPLICATION OF ETHICS

In order to apply principles of respect for individual human beings in the context of a hospital and its long-term residents we need to examine three aspects of their lives:
1. The patients' legal rights
2. The patients' physical environment
3. Behaviour of both staff and patients

The patients' legal rights

The law concerned with psychiatric patients has a dual function. Though one purpose is to protect the public from 'mentally disordered' people who exhibit violence, incorporated within the Mental Health Act, (1983) are a number of sections which give patients defined rights, designed for their freedom and protection. Although this was a great advance on earlier legislation, their status does not yet equate with that of citizens in the community and is inadequate in a number of respects. However, no doubt public opinion will continue to rectify such deficiencies and effect revisions in the form of amendments to the Mental Health Act.

Laws concerning welfare of patients in psychiatric hospitals mirror the attitude of a highly enlightened group of people within the community who hold certain views regarding ethical behaviour towards patients. However, there is no guarantee that such laws will always be upheld, despite the penalties prescribed for failure to implement any part of the Act. Even when all legal requirements are fulfilled, there is no legislation ensuring its requirements are carried out with such desirable qualities of conduct as respect and sincere feelings of warmth towards the patient. The ultimate responsibility for such standards of performance rests entirely with the people who directly care for patients, particularly those physically nearest to them, and when they do carry out their duties in accord with these high standards of conduct they do so as free agents.

Despite all adverse criticism, the Mental Health Act (1983), remains the patients' charter. When comparing present law with previous legislation few would challenge its claim to being more understanding of the needs and rights of psychiatric patients than its legal predecessors— the Lunacy Acts of 1890 and 1891, and the Mental Health Act 1959. Yet closer investigation of this comparison reveals a number of anomalies, not least of which is the considerable gap between legislators' intentions and the result of those intentions as they apply to long-term patients. There are many long-stay patients who are today completely unaware of the existence of such legislation, let alone have detailed knowledge of the relevant sections which personally apply to them. When one 'veteran' patient, for example, informed a newly appointed charge nurse he was going into town, he produced and proudly displayed his 'parole' card to prove he had the privilege. The charge nurse curiously examined the card for he remembered being told about 'parole' cards by a colleague with 30 years' service, but this was the first time he had ever seen one. He explained that such cards had been abandoned when the Mental Health Act, 1959 came into operation, and thus they were no longer necessary. The patient looked perplexed, but replaced the tattered card carefully in a plastic wallet, put it in his jacket pocket and left the ward with a puzzled expression.

Some patients are unable to understand anything more than a simple sentence, but those who are able to comprehend and to whom the main points of this law are explained, rarely react in a positive way. That they are no longer compulsorily detained and are now classified as 'informal' patients appears to have little impact on most patients' lives. They neither make demands for immediate discharge from hospital, as they might well have done in earlier days soon after admission to hospital, nor do they contemplate discharge as a remote possibility in the future.

The rigid restrictive rules applying to visitors of patients in mental hospitals have been swept aside, and visiting regulations are now more liberal than those existing in general hospitals. However, even allowing for the ravages of time, in terms of physical incapacity and possibly death of some of their relatives and friends, the tendency remains for visiting to decline proportionately with the patient's length of stay in hospital. This situation may be understandable when patients have been in hospital for 20 years or more, but a fall-off in visiting is noticeable soon after admission to hospital, and even more marked if the patient should be transferred to a long-stay ward. In a patient's case, absence does not make the heart grow fonder but leads to estrangement and the eventual severing of lifelines with the community.

Furthermore, long-stay patients tend to lack interest in voting and voicing their opinion on local and national affairs. This is a matter of great concern, but we suggest that a matter of greater importance is that they should first be actively encouraged to voice their opinion on matters affecting their personal lives on the wards in which they now live.

Voluntary organizations may act as advocates on behalf of these silent patients and be successful in influencing parliament to place further laws on the statute book, spelling out the patient's improved status in detail, but if the net result of such action fails to produce radical change in their life-style, such legislation will remain a hollow victory both for legislators and long-stay patients.

The formal introduction of laws, rules or regulations designed to bring a more liberal and humane influence into the lives of long-stay psychiatric patients is insufficient in itself to induce change. It needs to be followed up by some action, a set of procedures or a treatment, call it what you will, which transforms the idea into a meaningful reality for the patient. When we obey the letter of the law we do nothing more than perform the minimal action expected of us; when we implement the spirit and intention of the law we perform ethical conduct.

The patients' physical environment

The conditions in which patients live were surveyed in the chapter on institutionalization. The suggested modifications of the environment are not only practical steps towards treatment but have ethical implications as well. These modifications would be justified on ethical grounds alone, since the actions are an attempt to restore the dignity of the patients.

The initiation of major improvements in the physical environment of mental hospitals is a worthy venture and all people contributing to this cause deserve credit and honour for their work. However, history reveals that such changes are not solely dependent on the efforts of one person; they are not achieved without opposition, nor when finally achieved, do they produce instant beneficial results.

One of the outstanding personalities in psychiatric history was the physician Philippe Pinel, acknowledged as the man who removed chains from 40 patients in Bicetre Asylum. Less well known was the man who acted as his collaborator, Jean-Baptiste Pussin, a nurse who was referred to by Pinel as the 'Governor' (equivalent to today's Senior Nursing Officer in the hospital). Pinel started his labour of reformation in 1793 but was transferred to the Salpetrière institution before the change could be completed. It was left to Pussin and his nursing attendants to implement the reforms, which were finally achieved in 1798. These environmental changes were repeated at Salpetrière after Pussin was transferred there at Pinel's special request, but success was not achieved until 3 years later in 1801. This major event is often portrayed as a dramatic change which produced a favourable instant effect on the public and the 'liberated' patients. In truth it did neither, for the public remained antagonistic to the idea of unchaining these 'wild animals' and the patients, though freed from their iron fetters, were liberated only in the sense that they were now able to walk with attendant escort in the grounds of the institution with the sole restriction of their strait-jackets.

If such changes had little immediate benefit, there is now no doubt that this modification of the patients' circumstances was the first stage in paving the way for a more humanitarian attitude to mentally disordered patients, and it was the accomplishment of this change in policy which preceded a change of attitude. Once a change of attitude was established, the expectation of improvement in the patients' behaviour was raised, and in many cases improvement was realized.

The situations of yesterday have their modern counterpart. Similar attitudes exist in people who are emotionally resistant to change whatever the considered reform. There is no doubt that a great deal has been achieved over the years in the way of 'upgrading' the physical surroundings of the patients, within the limits of the financial resources available. Structural alterations, new furnishings and redecoration have all taken place, but not without struggle against the officials who eventually provided the means and the materials for the improvements. What is disconcerting is the reception given to these changes by some staff whose attitudes are revealed in such disparaging comments as 'A waste of time', 'A waste of money', 'They can't appreciate it', 'They'll ruin it in no time'. Unhappily, many of these adverse remarks are justified, for it is true many patients will misuse or fail to use some of the utilities provided and there is ample evidence on the wards to prove it. The criticism that all patients fail to notice and ignore the more aesthetic decorative features such as pictures, curtains, wallpaper, etc. is open to doubt. What is not justifiable is the tendency to group every patient in this problem area, for, although it may be true of many patients, it is by no means true of all. The first practical step we need to take is to identify the patients who fail to respond appropriately to these changes and direct our attention to them, by designing programmes which will help them to use the utilities appropriately and with skill.

One patient, who was transferred from a ward where he had a locker next to his dormitory bed to a ward where he had a single room with a fitted wardrobe, was easy to identify. After undressing and before getting into bed, his nightly routine was to roll his trousers tightly into a 'sausage' shape and place them inside his jacket, which he then buttoned up. He next folded his coat over, using the sleeves to tie his garments into a neat bundle which he placed underneath his bed. His shoes were then perched on top of the bundle like twin coronets resting on a velvet cushion.

This patient had been resident in the hospital for 23 years, his diagnosis was 'schizophrenia', but this behaviour was certainly no part of his psychotic symptoms. It was a learned behaviour directly attributable to the influence of the hospital environment, and the history of his 'odd' behaviour was not difficult to trace. In the early days of his admission, when conditions were more crowded, many patients did not have lockers for their clothing and possessions. Dormitory conditions were such that there was barely any room for a person to walk sideways between beds. One ingenious invention designed to overcome this problem was the fixing of a metal drawer underneath and at the foot of the bed where the patient could deposit his clothing before retiring.

Over the years and with rough handling, many of the clothing drawers deteriorated and became rusty; they no longer glided smoothly down the full length of the guides and often projected so far beyond the foot of the beds they became hazards. Thus the drawers were detached and placed on the floor *beneath* the beds and patients continued to use the drawers in their new location. When the patient population slowly decreased and the area of floor space between beds became noticeably large enough for bedside lockers to be introduced, the old-fashioned metal 'wardrobes' were sent to the scrap yard. Removal of the metal drawers and their replacement with bedside lockers did not, however, change the patients' behaviour. They continued to bundle their clothing and place it underneath their beds where the drawers *used* to be. They had been taught, one is tempted to say 'drilled', only too well.

Knowing and understanding the conditions in which people live or have lived in the past may help to explain some of the strange behaviours of long-stay patients. After 13 weeks of continuous treatment based on behavioural modification principles this particular patient *did* begin to use his wardrobe appropriately to store his clothes and did so without prompting from the nurses.

There is little doubt that environment does influence behaviour, but, when the environment is suddenly changed, it is unrealistic to expect immediate favourable responses from patients who have been deprived of the use of newly introduced facilities for many years. After all, the patients at Bicetre and Salpetrière who were chained to the walls like wild animals did not immediately become docile and amenable human beings when their chains were discarded. They had to re-learn more appropriate behaviour over a period of time.

Reviewing more recent historical examples in this country, we find similar illustrations of staff attitudes to change, involving responses of pessimism and forecasts of doom which rarely materialized. For example, when hospitals decided to introduce 'open' wards there was great fear expressed by staff that this venture would result in patients absconding from the hospital. While some patients did take advantage of this opportunity of freedom, many did not. In fact there was great difficulty in persuading most of them to leave the ward and walk in the grounds, a behaviour they had not performed for years without the benefit of a nurse escort. After a time they did step out of the ward and could be seen walking a circular route in the airing court, an identical path to one they used to travel when in a group under supervision of a watchful nurse.

When knives and forks were allowed to be used by long-stay patients in addition to spoons, resistance reared its ugly head again. Warnings that many fatalities would result fortunately fell on deaf ears and the consequences of this act were less dramatic. The main problem was to teach patients to use cutlery appropriately and to break their habit of using spoons for all types of food. The staff's fear lingered on in the ritual of counting the cutlery before distribution at mealtimes, and recounting before being put away. Not until this ritual was completed and all the utensils accounted for, were patients allowed to rise and leave their tables. The cutlery was then returned to its stout wooden box and ceremoniously locked by the nurse in charge. The final act completing this ceremony was to enter into the daily ward report book the number of utensils distributed and returned and present these record details to the nursing officer in charge.

There are numerous other examples which demonstrate this evolutionary cycle of change with its attitudes of fear, resistance and opposition then final acceptance. In retrospect it seems incredible that these events should have engendered such anxiety and conflict. It is tempting to speculate how long it would have been, if Pinel and Pussin had failed to achieve their aim of removing the shackles from the patients before another reformer came along and achieved success. 'Could such a distressful situation have continued for so long that it existed today?' We may well reply that such a situation would not be tolerated today, but when today's incidents and events have become tomorrow's history, will future generations comment on our attitudes and behaviour and also say, 'Such things could never happen now'?

Behaviour of staff and patients

To discuss behaviours of hospital patients in isolation from behaviours of nurses would inevitably result in presenting an unbalanced picture, for the relationship between their respective behaviours is so close.

Despite the accent which is usually placed on the *hidden mental processes* of psychotic patients, it is the bizarre, indecent or harmful *exhibited behaviours* which bring the patient to the immediate attention of other people and, dependent on the attitudes of these people, eventually bring them to hospital for treatment. The 'other people' initially involved may be members of the patient's own family, neighbours, the general public, social workers, doctors, police or members of the legal profession. However, it is nurses rather than doctors who finally have the greatest opportunity of social involvement with patients during their period of residence, and thus it is the nurse's attitudes and behaviours which have the greatest impact at this stage. Many behaviours patients display in public tend to elicit attitudes which result in emotions of fear or embarrassment rather than sympathy, for although society has a more enlightened view of mental illness it is not yet tolerant of odd behaviours which are unpredictable and for which there does not appear to be a rational explanation or an established cause. Few people would describe physical violence, shouting of obscenities, incontinence of urine or continuous incomprehensible talk as endearing behaviours; yet psychiatric nurses are expected to understand, to tolerate and to give tender loving care to the very people who exhibit behaviours which produce feelings of revulsion and animosity in their fellow citizens. If we are to regard patients as people we must also regard *nurses* as people and consider the difficulties and problems involved in playing these dual conflicting roles as ordinary members of the public and as nurses in the equally 'real-life' situation of the psychiatric hospital.

ETHICAL DILEMMAS

Our attitudes are shaped by many factors during the course of our life. Our parents, teachers, living conditions, economic situation and religion, all help to influence and form our views, opinions and prejudices about a vast range of subjects concerning people and events. Indeed, it is these factors which may very well have influenced our entry into our present employment, although we may prefer to think it is the result of free choice. In private life it is possible for nurses to avoid certain people and situations that arouse disturbing emotions; but as nurses in the hospital work situation it is not. Nursing concerns the head and the heart, and this balance of the combined intellect and the emotions determine the quality of care which is given to the patient. What we think and how strongly we think about the actions to take in specific situations, and the techniques we use to cope with some of the ethical dilemmas which may arise when confronted with potentially inflammatory circumstances are important aspects worthy of consideration.

We all tend to have views on controversial topics such as abortion, sterilization of male sexual offenders or mentally retarded and sexually precocious adolescent girls, and the maintenance of life by mechanical means of severely brain-damaged and unconscious people. Our degree of concern about any of these topics tends to equate with the amount of past personal involvement in such situations during the course of our life. As a psychiatric nurse working in hospital it is highly unlikely we would be involved in making decisions about such delicate matters, although we may occasionally come into contact with patients who have been or are the centre of such controversial problems.

The ethical dilemmas we may find ourselves involved in may seem less controversial than these topics, but the consequences of our behaviour can have major significance for the patient and ourselves. For example, it is likely we have opinions about 'informal' patients who are considered incapable of looking after themselves and who leave the hospital without knowledge or permission of the nurses on the ward. On the one hand, 'informal' patients have the legal right to freedom of movement to enter or leave hospital without restriction and, on the other hand, nurses have the moral responsibility to care for them and see they come to no harm. What is the right action to take in these circumstances? Whether a nurse chooses either the legal or moral approach, the result could be equally disastrous for herself and her patients. The consequences of the patient's behaviour may result in complaints from the public, or ultimately his death; the consequences for the nurse may be adverse criticism of her capabilities from senior staff, or attendance at a coroner's inquest with more menacing implications which may jeopardize her career. Under these circumstances it may sound reasonable to perform the actions which involve the least risk to both patient and nurse but, unfortunately, when we consider these actions in detail we find they are also antitherapeutic.

24-hour constant surveillance. Due to shortage of staff this is difficult to implement in most cases. It is also a retrograde step insofar as the patient may be deprived of the opportunity of learning to cope with life outside the hospital and attain any privacy or degree of independence. It is hardly a morale booster for nurses undertaking this duty.

Increase drug dosage. This is considered by many people as an unethical measure, for though it may produce satisfactory results in reducing hyperactivity sufficient to prevent the patient going absent from the ward it may also hinder any treatment programmes required to improve or maintain other behaviours.

Patients wear pyjamas and dressing gown. This allows the patient a greater degree of freedom on the ward and also makes it easy to identify him if he passes the hospital boundary. However, if the patient has problems relating to dressing or appearance, remedial programmes must remain in abeyance. Visits to outside social functions are restricted and he may also be barred from attending occupational or industrial units with consequent loss of income. This particular approach to the problem does not accord with 'preserving the patient's dignity'.

Transfer to locked ward. This eliminates the need for any of the previous actions and relieves the staff on the 'open' ward of worrying responsibilities. The patient may now have the freedom of the ward, maintain his dignity and retain his contact with all possible work and social activities even though he does so as a member of a nurse-escorted group. A disadvantage is that any nurse–patient relationships established on his previous ward are destroyed, but the main questionable point is the legality of detaining an 'informal' patient in a closed environment because he absents himself from hospital.

The immediate convenience of some of these modes of action probably accounts for their frequent use. The major criticisms arise when (1) no provision is made to investigate the reasons for the patient's absences, (2) when there is no planned systematic procedure to determine how long the adopted method should last, and (3) when no plans are prepared to assist the patient to overcome the inadequacies which constitute the main problem.

Unless a more structured approach to the problem is organized at ward level, staff tend to regard the patient as one who represents a constant threat to disrupt the routine of the ward and cause inconvenience to nurses. This negative attitude toward the patient, which can hardly be regarded as a foundation for the establishment of a good relationship, usually results in hesitancy and reluctance to terminate any of the actions taken for fear of a resumption of the patient's behaviour of absence without leave. Thus, the nurse responsible for initiating these procedures demonstrates little confidence in the efficacy of these methods either as short-term measures or long-term remedial treatments, and the patient is restricted for an indeterminate and usually extended period of time which may only elapse at the whim of the nurse in charge or take place by accident rather than design.

Further situations can be cited which produce antagonistic results depending on the action taken. One example is the need to give patients maximum privacy, particularly when bathing. This conflicts with a hospital rule which decrees no patient should be left in the bathroom without a nurse being present. Programmes which promote independence in patients are regarded as worthy aims deserving encouragement, but regulations which require nurses to run water and test temperatures for *all* patients before they enter the bath, are incompatible with patient independence in this self-care activity.

On many wards there are a number of elderly patients who may be capable of walking short distances but whose sense of balance is so faulty they are always at risk of falling on the floor and possibly breaking a limb. Should the nurse insist in placing such a patient 'at risk' in a geriatric chair for his own protection? Suppose the patient continues to be restless in the geriatric chair and is in danger of overturning it, is the nurse justified in putting the patient to bed to prevent even more serious injury? If the patient maintains this restlessness in bed, should cot-sides be used or medication suggested to the doctor in charge?

Most nurses will have experienced similar problematic situations and their decision will have been primarily concerned with preventing the patient from harming himself, although the consequences of these dangers, such as having to call the doctor, arrange an ambulance for the patient's admission to the casualty department for X-rays, the writing of accident reports, notification of relatives and possible future accusations of neglect that may be levelled against the staff, are never completely absent from mind. From the patient's point of view, such actions may be regarded as infringements of his basic liberty—the freedom to walk about—and even if he is incapable of verbally expressing it, he will often forcibly communicate the message by exhibiting other behaviours of an 'unco-operative' nature.

The 'care and protection' ideal versus the 'promotion and mainten-ance of basic freedoms' concept is not easy to resolve. It appears that much of the nurses' behaviour at work in hospital is governed by four factors: (1) the law, (2) hospital regulations, (3) ward rules and

(4) ethical considerations. Where the strength of regard and respect for all these categories of influence is equal but in particular circumstances their aims conflict, as when regulations restrict the operation of treatment, then the nurse concerned must make a personal decision based on what is considered the most important factor operating at that time in that situation. Unfortunately, of these four factors, ethical considerations may be the one most likely to suffer, especially when it involves treatments which prove difficult to implement because of the restrictions of existing rules and regulations. This dilemma gives rise to different types of nurse who attempt to solve the problem or come to terms with it in various ways:

The overzealous nurse who may well risk a clash with the law or hospital regulations if ethical reasons are personally considered to have priority. Often regarded as an idealist, she is one of the rare breed of reformers and usually an individualist who finds it difficult to function in a team unless invested with authority to lead the team. She may try to alter rules or even make a personal interpretation of the law before taking action, but when attempts at changing regulations fail to result in immediate success she is intolerant of delay and likely to proceed with behaviours which provoke higher authority. In the long term this type of nurse rarely achieves any desired aims. It is unlikely there will ever be another 'Florence Nightingale'.

The overcautious nurse who usually resolves any ethical dilemmas by choosing the action least likely to arouse controversy. Though often stated to have a healthy respect for law and order, and a consideration for patients, she may be described by others as a dull conformist whose main concern is self-preservation. Unlike the former type of nurse, she will participate in procedures of therapeutic change if inaugurated and monitored by others of higher authority but rarely attempts even minor changes on her own initiative, despite official encouragement.

Few nurses will recognize themselves in either of these categories for they are extremes—exaggerated examples drawn for the purpose of illustration. However, most nurses have traces of all these characteristics, and it is with these that the responsibility for favourable changes within the hospital rest. While no rational person would advocate flouting the law, some hospital regulations and ward rules are capable of being amended to become more flexible in circumstances where therapeutic procedures are proposed. When proposals for modification are presented in a logical rather than emotional manner to those capable of amending the rules, then a successful outcome which paves the way for intended treatment is more likely. In order to ensure a maximum chance of success for any proposed treatment programme, all staff on the ward need to understand the rationale of any planned procedure so that they may co-ordinate their attitudes and behaviour and avoid unilateral actions which will confuse the patient.

When we consider the very essence of life as consisting of a number of risks, it is both irrational to think and unethical to attempt to provide a 100% perpetual protective environment for our long-stay patients. We need to be a little more adventurous in our approach to patients' problems in order to gradually give them back responsibility for their own behaviour. Though this adventurous approach does involve a minor element of risk, it is a carefully calculated one, based on knowledge of the principles of behavioural treatment and always performed with offical approval and constantly open to public investigation.

CRITICISM OF BEHAVIOURAL TREATMENT

We consider behavioural treatment is in little need of defence against attacks from its critics who frequently revile its procedures on ethical grounds; for, in retrospect, the major problems concerning long-stay patients in hospitals or other residential settings which have triggered the need for official inquiries have rarely been due to the introduction of such treatments, but rather to the lack of them.

Nevertheless, it would be unwise not to counteract some of the more emotive accusations and misinterpretations with objective explanations, not so much for the purpose of defence, but for the reason of providing information and knowledge to those who retain a genuine and more objective interest in this subject. Some common statements of critical condemnation are examined below.

'Behavioural treatment is an inhuman and degrading form of treatment'

No one seriously suggests that the majority of treatments are pleasant experiences, whether the treatment be a surgical operation, a course of intramuscular injections, electroconvulsive therapy or a series of psychoanalytical sessions. All these treatments possess a common factor representing some form of assault on the body or disturbance to the mind, and in this context all treatments can be equally described as degrading.

Sometimes an illness itself is regarded as degrading by the community, especially those diseases which are known to be infectious, including syphilis and tuberculosis. When treatment involves some form of physical and social isolation, the feeling of rejection and contamination is strengthened. Even mental illnesses still retain an element of social stigma despite the lack of any evidence to justify this attitude. The effect on the sufferer can be shattering when both the illness and nature of assistance given is thought of as degrading and an affront to his dignity; but help can never be regarded as inhuman.

Not to attempt treatment, not to give assistance—*this* is inhuman. Like other forms of treatment, behaviour therapy is a treatment which concentrates on and attempts to restore the patient to a functional level as near as possible to that which existed prior to his illness, and therefore its motives are based on firm humanitarian principles—to relieve suffering. Failure to use this form of treatment in a situation which may enable an individual to improve the quality of his life would amount to an act of neglect—the very antithesis of humanitarianism. Few actions could be regarded as more undignified and degrading to an adult human being than continuing to provide him with assistance and organizing the details of his life when he may have the potential to perform these activities for himself.

There are problem areas for which there are no alternative treatments to behavioural treatment, particularly those behaviour problems closely associated with the effects of institutionalization. Though behavioural treatments do involve stress factors for the patient, they are carefully graduated ones, carefully 'tailored' to the individual patient's capacity and are less unpleasant and certainly less dangerous than many other forms of treatment.

'I have no quarrel with its motives but rather its methods'

The critic now changes the direction of his attack; the hostility is refocused from the general to the particular and concentrates on specific methods used in the individual programmes.

'For example, an undue amount of control is used which restricts the patient's freedom'

No therapist can conduct a treatment programme without some form of control. In drug therapy, no one would seriously suggest the type of drug, the amount, or the frequency of administration should be left to the discretion of each individual nurse on duty or the whim of the patient. Such irresponsible conduct would lead to ineffective or dangerous consequences. The doctor writes the prescription on a treatment card, determines the drug, the dosage, times of administration and delegates the responsibility of carrying out his instructions to nurses. Each nurse becomes responsible for ensuring the patient takes the right drug in the correct dosage at the instructed times. Observation by nurses of the patient's reactions to the drug are conveyed to the doctor who will review treatment on the basis of these observations and his own experience. When the patient is ready for discharge but is required to continue drug treatment, the doctor has to judge and decide if the patient is capable of being responsible for controlling his own drug administration. Thus treatment starts with rigid control, and as the responses to treatment become effective and stabilized any continuation of treatment is eventually handed over to the patient, who is freed of the restrictions imposed by the very nature of his illness and the institution where treatment took place.

Similarly with behavioural treatments; rigid control is essential in the early stages to ensure appropriate behaviours are reinforced immediately after they occur and inappropriate behaviours are never reinforced. Like the drugs, reinforcers are under the control of the people who treat the patient. The treatment programme is written in the form of instructions and describes the actions nurses should take in specific circumstances, all the staff following the same instructions written on the treatment chart in the same way they follow instructions written on a patient's medicine card. Observations and responses to treatment are charted and considered when reviewing the patient's treatment. As soon as treatment results in improvement of the patient's behavioural problem, he is informed of his favourable progress and attempts are made to involve him in his own treatment to encourage him to further improve or maintain his behaviour. As in the example of drug therapy, rigid control is essential at the start of treatment, with improvement determining onset of relaxation of control, until the patient finally takes over complete responsibility for his own behaviour. One important aspect of behavioural treatment which must be emphasized is that all procedures should be performed in a firm but friendly personal manner, not only for ethical reasons but also because this friendly relationship often determines the course of the treatment.

The main restriction on the freedom of the untreated psychiatric patient stems from his own inappropriate, excessive or deficient behaviours. The aim of behavioural treatment is to remedy this situation by teaching him appropriate social skills and provide suitable environments in which he can practise those skills, until the control exercised is that of the patient himself and the only other restrictions which remain are those imposed by the society in which he lives.

Without treatment the patient will still be able to retain his freedom, but it will be a freedom to indulge in odd behaviours which restrict him to hospital for possibly the rest of his life. Whether such indulgences represent a responsible conscious decision by the patient is open to grave doubt. That a patient should be allowed this kind of freedom is an ethical question to which the answer should *not* be in doubt.

In summary of the topic of ethics, one question remains to be answered: is there a special relationship between ethics and behavioural treatment?

One point of view is that behavioural treatment has no greater relevance to ethics than that of other forms of treatment. As far as nurses are concerned, the topic of ethics is presented as a primary subject very early in nurse training and 'pops up' at frequent intervals throughout the course syllabus, particularly when discussing patient's privacy, confidentiality and comfort. In view of this fact, there does not appear to be any need to unduly emphasize the importance of ethics by presenting it as a separate subject. This opinion may be summarized by stating that the conduct of behavioural treatments simply involve nothing more than the same high professional standards as those required for other forms of treatment.

An alternative point of view, however, is of ethics occupying a *unique* position in connection with the practice of behavioural treatment, and its importance needs to be stressed for two reasons.

1. NURSE–PATIENT RELATIONSHIPS ARE AN INTEGRAL PART OF TREATMENT

Unlike drug therapy or treatments which do not completely rely on the patient's conscious personal involvement for their success, behavioural treatment is positively dependent on it.

Establishing and maintaining a good relationship between patient and nurse is, therefore, regarded as a 'key' element in the success of behavioural treatment. The patient's motivation and involvement in his own treatment are considered to be important factors which can only be achieved when behavioural techniques and procedures are based upon a sincere and friendly relationship with the patient. Techniques which involve a detached attitude, or procedures which possess aversive features cannot establish desirable relationships.

It is extremely important that practitioners of behavioural treatment become aware of the effect of their own attitudes, motives and behaviour on the behaviour of their patients, and the degree to which it influences results of treatment. This knowledge and its application represents a considerable proportion of the therapist's skill. On this evidence, it is beyond doubt that behavioural treatment *has* a special relationship with ethics because the success of treatment depends a great deal on the skill of the therapist in practising a high standard of conduct.

2. THE NEED TO SPREAD BEHAVIOURAL TREATMENT

Behavioural treatments which result in improvement of a patient's behaviour need to be progressively generalized to a variety of places within the hospital and eventually, for selected high-level patients, extended into the community outside the hospital. To limit treatment within the confines of one area would be tantamount to denying the patient complete treatment—a highly unethical situation.

It is the hospital administrators and professional workers within the hospital, such as social workers and disablement resettlement officers, who can establish official links with statutory and voluntary services, giving the patient access to accommodation and employment which complete the final links in the chain of rehabilitation. Before giving official approval to any major changes in the organizational structure of the hospital, responsible officials will understandably require evidence to justify these changes, particularly when the treatment may be considered controversial.

The introduction of any new form of treatment into a hospital is likely to come under keen scrutiny by all staff working in that hospital. When nurses possess the major responsibility for its design and operation, one can be certain that such a revolutionary innovation will be examined more critically. An investigation into the operation of behavioural treatments should be welcomed by all people working in this specialty, for it provides an opportunity to broadcast not only the theory and practice of the treatment, but also the philosophy which lies behind the treatment. Senior medical, nursing and administration officers are justifiably concerned about the protection of the patient as well as the reputation of the hospital, and the need to ensure the methods of treatment do not contravene hospital policy, unduly restrict freedom, or interfere with the legal rights of patients.

The skill of those using behavioural treatment is based on a foundation of ethical conduct. As long as they maintain a vigilant and critical attitude to their work and behaviour, rejecting any aspect which may conflict with those high standards, they will be in a strong position to answer adverse criticism and present their case with confidence, not only to the official representatives of the hospital but also to the community beyond the hospital with resulting benefit to the patient.

SECTION III
MEASURING BEHAVIOUR

Chapter 8

NORMAL BEHAVIOUR

All the actions we perform every day of our lives can be summarized in one word—behaviour. The two main qualities of behaviour are termed 'normal' and 'abnormal', but the kinds of behaviour which make up these qualities are often a matter of personal opinion. We are more likely to agree with each other that a particular behaviour is abnormal when we witness it in an extreme form. When extreme forms of behaviour are absent, we are more likely to assume normal behaviour is present. Many behaviours, however, fail to fit neatly into either of these categories and may become the subject of disagreement. In most cases these differences of opinion have little importance beyond providing a brief period of entertaining discussion.

When the behaviour under discussion raises doubts about a person's mental stability and responsibility for his actions, or results in expressions of concern for his welfare or the welfare of other people, then personal opinions do matter. They matter because they have important consequences for the individual concerned and, in these circumstances, differences of opinion need to be urgently resolved.

Society usually delegates the responsibilities of making final judgements about human behaviour to specialists, people trained and experienced in the areas of law, medicine and psychiatry. It is these specialists who investigate, make judgements and decide, or recommend, the course of action to be taken. They do not, however, make these decisions alone. In turn, they depend upon the collaboration of their colleagues who form members of a team and, in the areas of medicine and psychiatry, nurses are important members of that team. Because nurses are with patients for longer periods of time than other professions, they have greater opportunities of observing patients' behaviour in a variety of situations. It is important, therefore, that reports of their observations are as fair to the patient as possible and meaningful to those who read them.

We are mainly concerned with the group of abnormal behaviours classified as 'psychiatric disorders' and need to have understanding of these conditions. We must be equally concerned and have understanding of the standards of conduct which constitute *normal* behaviour for three important reasons.

1. *Diagnosis*

Abnormal behaviour can only be diagnosed when it is compared with an agreed standard of behaviour defined as normal. It is this standard which represents a unit of measurement which helps to assess the patient's behaviour and results in a diagnosis.

Unfortunately, no textbook can give a precise definition of normal behaviour and can only offer guidelines in deciding its quality and range. It is important we investigate and explore the subject of normal behaviour if we are to use it as an instrument of measurement, for without an understanding of normal behaviour a diagnosis of abnormal behaviour can never be fairly made.

2. *Treatment*

Normality is the ultimate target of all treatment. It is as well to keep this goal in mind when considering forms of measuring behavioural changes which take place during the course of treatment. It is a more optimistic approach to measure the quantity and quality of normal behaviour the patient can perform rather than dwell on the presence or absence of his abnormal behaviours. When diagnosing a patient's abnormal behaviour, our intention is to find out the severity of his problem by comparing his behaviour with a standard of normal behaviour. In other words. 'How *bad* is he?' During treatment we want to know, 'How *well* is he?'

3. *Recovery*

If we regard recovery as the highest level of normal behaviour a patient can reach and maintain, then this level of improvement can be measured in several ways. One approach involves comparing his behaviour before treatment with his existing behaviour. Another way is to compare his improved level of behaviour with the behaviour of other people—people who are regarded as being well and normal. Comparing a patient's behaviour before and after treatment may produce some exceedingly favourable results, particularly in the case of a patient who had severe behavioural problems to begin with. Yet, even with this highly dramatic improvement in such a patient, the level of his improvement may fall considerably short of what most of us would regard as normal behaviour.

A third and more meaningful way to find out if a patient has reached a state of recovery would be to compare his present behaviour with his behaviour *before* he became ill. That is, to discover his own individual standard of normality. Patients who have been in hospital for a relatively short period are often able to supply this information themselves with relatives being able to fill in the gaps. A complete set of behaviours may result which gives the therapist a good idea of the 'normality' standard of that particular patient. It is unfortunate that patients who have spent many years living in hospital are usually less articulate and less reliable in the information they give to the therapist. When relatives are not readily available to check statements the patient gives or to give additional information, a long-term patient's standard of normality can rarely be verified. Examination of the case notes of a long-term patient for these important details is rarely successful.

We may, therefore, have to rely more on the former two methods of assessment, i.e. compare the patient's behaviour before treatment with his existing level of improved behaviour, and compare his improved level of behaviour with that of the normal behaviour of other people.

Accepting this emphasis on the importance of normal behaviour, we are still left with the question, 'What is normal behaviour?' Normal behaviour means, of course, all the things you and I do. This definition is quite popular, for we do tend to think of ourselves as examples of normality. Even so, few of us would deny we do occasionally act a little 'odd'. A degree of abnormality in certain circumstances is often quite acceptable and maybe expected. For example, if we won a first dividend of £100,000 on a football pool and did not depart from our normal pattern of behaviour in some way, people would think it decidedly odd.

We are living in a period of time which has been labelled 'the permissive society'. Many behaviours we regarded as unacceptable 10 or more years ago, now come into the range of normal behaviour. In the not-so-distant past, a person who made persistent announcements about 'men flying to the moon', would have been described as a lunatic. Today it is a perfectly acceptable statement. Fact has now caught up with some science fiction.

It appears that any attempt to define 'normal' behaviour must take into account a great number of factors, including scientific achievement as well as the prevailing attitudes of society. We must learn to constantly review and revise our personal ideas of normality, because standards of normal behaviour are always in the process of change. If we are to use our personal standards of normality as measuring instruments to be employed in diagnosis and treatment, we must be sure they are frequently calibrated against the current attitudes and views of other people and in harmony with them.

There are, of course, many other factors to take into account. Take the situation of a lady who decided to do some shopping. After collecting her shopping bag and money, she stepped out of the house and closed the door behind her. She walked down the path, but before entering the street she suddenly wondered if she had locked the door. In order to make sure, she returned to the house and tried to open the door, and as it would not open, it was obviously locked. Her behaviour was that of a perfectly normal person. Setting off down the garden path she stopped once more and returned to the house door and performed the same behaviour. Appearing to be satisfied she set off once more on her shopping expedition. After all, the lady was just 'security-minded'.

When she had performed this behaviour 124 times, her neighbour, looking through the curtains in the house opposite, decided there was something abnormal about this behaviour. It appears that a perfectly normal behaviour can become abnormal when it is practised with *excessive frequency*.

Removing our clothing in order to prepare for a medical examination by a doctor is a perfectly normal behaviour. Getting completely undressed before meeting other people in a nudist camp is a perfectly normal behaviour. Taking off all your clothes when shopping in the city centre—that is indecent! When measuring normal behaviour, we must take into account not only the behaviour itself, but also the *place in which it occurs*.

Two women were overheard talking to each other on a bus:
'How's your Jimmy getting on, has he started to talk yet?'
'Oh yes, he's going on fine thank you', replied her companion. 'He now says 'Mummy', 'Daddy' and 'ta.'
'That's nice, how old is he now?'
'He'll be 24 years old next Monday.'

In this case, one may surmise that her son was either mentally retarded from birth, or had made a slight recovery from some serious brain damage. Whatever the circumstances, the *age* of the person performing the behaviour must be taken into consideration when assessing a person's normal standard of behaviour.

A detailed explanation of Einstein's theory of relativity given by a university graduate may be accepted as normal behaviour. A similar behaviour by an 8-year-old child will definitely not be regarded as normal. Society labels outstanding attainments, which are far above the level achieved by the majority of the population, as 'genius'.

Extremely high as well as a low level of achievement may be regarded as abnormal behaviour. When attempting to decide normal behaviour between these extremes, one must know, not only the age of the person concerned but also the level of *training and education* he has received.

The clothing a person wears, as well as the manner it is worn, may be a manifestation of normal or abnormal behaviour. Wearing an Elizabethan costume may be normal behaviour if it is worn on a stage as a character in a play, at a fancy-dress ball, or a 'pop' concert. If such apparel is worn consistently when going to work at the factory, office or hospital, it may lead the wearer into some pretty tricky situations. These are obvious examples of the importance of looking at the place the behaviour occurs before deciding into which category it falls.

There is, however, the aspect of fashion to consider. A new garment, or a radical change in style of an existing item of clothing, must be accepted by the majority of people before it becomes fashionable. This change does not happen overnight. A minority of individuals wearing these styles are needed to start and lead a campaign of change. At this stage, individuals wearing the new style attract the attention of other people because their dress is so different from everyone else's. When the number of people wearing the new-style clothing increases to the point where they become the majority of the population, it is those people *not* wearing that particular style who become noticeable.

It is as well to remember that many long-term patients entered hospital with 'fashionable' clothing, some of which may be still in good condition. To go out in public and wear it today would identify them as 'odd'. Many of them have lost touch with the outside world and need to be re-acquainted with not only the fashion of clothing, but also other fashions connected with appearances, such as hair length and style.

Current styles and fashions represent a standard of normality in dress behaviour and play an important part in the areas of work and social activities. How far people wander from this standard can be regarded as a measurement of their degree of abnormal dress behaviour.

A person wearing 'normal' clothing can sometimes appear bizarre to other people. One man was repeatedly fined in a court of law because of his insistence on wearing a form of headwear normal to him but uncommon to the people in the community in which he lived. He was charged with failing to wear a crash helmet whilst driving a motor-bike. This man was a member of the Sikh religion and wore a turban, stating it was against his faith to remove his turban in public. As he found it impossible to wear a crash helmet and his turban at the same time, and because he needed his motor cycle to get to his work, he continued to be repeatedly charged for this offence by the police. The charges stopped when the law was amended to allow members of the Sikh faith to wear turbans in these circumstances. When assessing normal behaviour we must know the *cultural background* of a person before we interpret his behaviour as abnormal.

We have reviewed some aspects worth considering when trying to identify normal behaviour. In summary, they include:

Frequency of performance.
Location in which behaviour is performed.

Consideration of current fashions.

Awareness of changing standards.

Knowing and understanding the different cultural backgrounds of people.

There are many words used in our every day language which describe normal and abnormal behaviour:

Normal behaviour. Natural, ordinary, standard, typical, usual, sensible, common, average.

Abnormal behaviour. Silly, odd, eccentric, inappropriate, idiotic, insane, extraordinary, peculiar, strange, mad, lunatic, uncommon, deranged, disordered.

These words also have different strengths of meaning which are particularly noticeable under the heading of 'abnormal behaviour'. For example, the strength of 'silly' and 'odd' are usually regarded as weaker than 'insane' and 'lunatic'.

Generally accepted words describing different types of abnormal behaviour are:

Asocial. Socially embarrassing or offensive acts to other people, not amounting to physical violence. Commonly described as bad manners or rude behaviour. Deliberately avoiding other people in social contact. Socially withdrawn.

Antisocial. Behaviours which constitute criminal acts.

Pathological. Behaviours which are due to organic causes (e.g. brain damage, metabolic and circulatory disorders etc.)

Psychopathological. Behaviours not due to any known and proved organic cause. These are often called 'functional', and psychiatric text books usually sub-divide them into psychoses and neuroses. A third category of psychiatric problem is classified as socio-pathic or psychopathic personalities.

Between each classification there is a 'grey' area in which it is difficult to decide the category to which the behaviour belongs. The behaviours of long-term resident patients consist of a mixture of normal and abnormal behaviours, and the majority of patients have more normal behaviours in their repertoire than abnormal ones.

Many behavioural responses of patients would be accepted in the community outside the hospital, but because they occur within the walls of a psychiatric hospital, staff often interpret them as being due to the patient's psychiatric condition. 'After all, they are not here for nothing', is a statement often made by staff to justify their interpretation of most 'disruptive' behaviour of patients.

The last place to look for examples of normal behaviour is a psychiatric hospital. Not because it rarely exists, but because our familiarity with patients' behaviour and the environment in which they take place, clouds our judgement in distinguishing one type of behaviour from another. We, as well as the public, expect abnormal rather than normal behaviour to occur more frequently in a psychiatric hospital. Our expectations are frequently justified. All staff involved in treatment must eventually agree on two standards of normality: the common standard applicable to the society in which we live, and secondly, an agreed standard of normality for the individual patient. These standards represent the final targets of treatment.

Chapter 9

MEASURING AND RECORDING BEHAVIOUR

Whenever treatment is being carried out, records of the techniques used and the patient's response are always monitored in some way. These are of value to those conducting the treatment because the permanent record provides regular information on the patient's progress, and may indicate what the next steps in treatment might be.

The alternative to keeping records is to rely on memory with its inaccuracy of recall. Man's recall of events is affected both by the gradual fading of details with time and influence of personal bias and feeling. Consequently a record which is not susceptible to the same changes with time or circumstances must be of greater accuracy.

The daily duties of a nurse often involve recording events related to patients' treatment. We spend time, for example, marking in medicine cards and filling in TPR (temperature, pulse, respiration) charts. We may even record our own behaviour, as when filling in time sheets and leave forms. However the behaviour of long-stay patients is often not recorded with the same degree of care. Key events and incidents are written down in the nurses' notes or case notes, but are often difficult to evaluate and compare because of the poverty of the information, the sporadic entries and the style of recording.

Written records are only useful where the behaviour is accurately described and regular entries are made. Words such as 'disturbed' and 'comfortable' are open to wide interpretation because they are opinions not facts. Statements like, 'He put his fist through the window during O.T.' and, 'He said "hello" when I arrived this morning' are more precise because they describe only what actually happened. Written reports are particularly useful in keeping records of those behaviours which happen infrequently or occur in unusual circumstances.

In recording more frequent events, making statements such as, 'He is often seen pacing' or 'He is sometimes verbally aggressive' are inadequate. What does 'often' and 'sometimes' mean? Since behaviour can be 'seen' it can be measured. 'Sometimes' in this case could mean four times a day. To state, 'He was verbally aggressive four times today' gives a much more precise and accurate statement about the patient's behaviour because it eliminates any ambiguity that could arise through people interpreting 'sometimes' in different ways.

Since behaviour modification is concerned with changing the behaviour of a patient, measurements of his behaviour must be collected in a standard way and presented so his progress can be clearly determined, and communicated to others.

WAYS OF MEASURING BEHAVIOUR

There are four commonly used methods of measuring behaviour, each giving a different type of information. These are:

Counting—measures the frequency of a behaviour.
Timing—measures the duration of a behaviour.
Checking—measures the ability to perform a behaviour.
Rating—measures the quality of a behaviour.

Counting

When a patient does something a varying number of times a day, the simplest way of measuring it, is to *count*. Where a patient's problem behaviour is incontinence for example, counting the number of times he is 'wet' each day, gives a measure of the extent of his problem. Counting answers such questions as 'How frequently does a patient bang his head?' and 'How often does the patient wash his hands?'

The length of time needed to observe a patient depends on the behaviour in question. Thus if the behaviour occurs infrequently such as absconding from the ward or incontinence, each occurrence could be recorded whenever it happened throughout the day. Where behaviour occurs much more frequently, possibly in the case of a patient hitting himself, recording each event would be extremely time consuming for the nurse. However, it is possible to obtain a good idea of what a patient is like by taking a careful sample of his behaviour by using a *time sampling* technique. Time sampling involves observing the patient for a standard period of time at intervals spaced throughout the day, so for example we might observe him six times a day, for 5 minutes each time with an hour's interval between each observation. By altering the time at which the samples are taken in consecutive days an overall picture of the patient's behaviour can be accurately built up.

Timing

When a behaviour becomes a problem because of the length of time it takes to perform, the most appropriate way to measure it, is by *timing*. Timing answers such questions as, 'How long does it take a patient to dress in the morning?' and, 'How long does it take a patient to sweep the corridor?'

On most occasions a watch with a sweep second hand is adequate, but in a situation where the behaviour to be measured exhibits itself in short phases, a stopwatch may be necessary. A stopwatch would be needed for example to accurately measure how much a patient talked in a 30-minute discussion group, for his utterances would occur in short bursts, at irregular intervals.

Where a behaviour occurs quite frequently, as in pacing and talking to self, and we need to find out how long a patient indulges in such behaviours, time sampling may again be used. Here the observer times how long the behaviour occurs in perhaps 10-minute samples spaced throughout the day.

The length of a sample should depend on the rate at which the behaviour occurs. From *Fig.* 1 we can see that where behaviour occurs at a very high rate, such as smacking lips, the length of the sample may be as small as 2 minutes, but where the behaviour occurs less frequently the sample will be longer. Twenty minutes limits the length as after this the attention of the observer begins to wane.

In deciding on the number of samples to take, we need to consider the length of the sample. We have to keep in mind that the greater the number of samples taken a day the more reliable will be the results, but also that a greater burden is put on staff taking the measurements. When the length of a sample is short, say 2 minutes, a number of samples may be taken in quick succession as in *Fig.* 1, allowing for a short period in between to record the results, but where the length of a sample is long, the interval between samples needs to be greater.

There is a further time sampling technique which when applied correctly can give an accurate measure of a patient's behaviour. This involves taking a number of split-second observations of the patient and noting whether at these moments he was or was not performing the particular behaviour in question. Thus, if we required a measure of how often a patient talked to himself, we might decide to take an observation each half hour. We would then take one look at the patient at each specified time and note whether he was engaged in the behaviour or not. Such a sampling technique can obviously only be of assistance where the behaviour occurs reasonably frequently, but where these conditions are met, a reasonable picture of the patient's behaviour can be built up.

Checking

Checking involves observing a patient to see if a certain behaviour occurs or does not occur at that time. It therefore requires a simple yes–no decision from the observer, who by collating data on a number of similar checks, can measure the extent to which a patient performs a particular behaviour. Such questions as, 'Does a patient regularly get up before 7·15 in the morning?' can thus be answered.

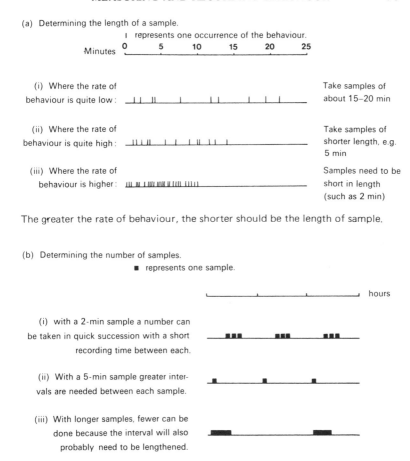

(a) Determining the length of a sample.

ı represents one occurrence of the behaviour.

Minutes 0   5   10   15   20   25

(i) Where the rate of
behaviour is quite low :   Take samples of
about 15–20 min

(ii) Where the rate of
behaviour is quite high :   Take samples of
shorter length, e.g.
5 min

(iii) Where the rate of
behaviour is higher :   Samples need to be
short in length
(such as 2 min)

The greater the rate of behaviour, the shorter should be the length of sample.

(b) Determining the number of samples.

■ represents one sample.

                                        hours

(i) with a 2-min sample a number can
be taken in quick succession with a short
recording time between each.

(ii) With a 5-min sample greater intervals are needed between each sample.

(iii) With longer samples, fewer can be
done because the interval will also
probably need to be lengthened.

The longer the sample the greater the need for length of interval between samples, so fewer samples can be taken.

Fig. 1. Time sampling.

When a number of related items are put together, they form a checklist as in *Fig.* 2. This is a convenient method for measuring the state or ability of a patient in, for example, his appearance, initiative, or work performance.

Where we need to have more detailed information about a patient's clothing, for example, and want to know more than whether the patient is wearing shoes or not but also whether the shoes are clean and whether

Patient's name _				
✓ Satisfactory				
✗ Unsatisfactory or Not present				
N/A Unrateable				
	Date			
1. Hair neat				
2. Face clean				
3. Absence of facial hair				
4. Dress clean				
5. Dress fastened properly				
6. Hands and nails clean				
7. Tights or stockings on				
8. Both shoes on				

Fig. 2. Example of part of a checklist for measuring the appearance of a female patient.

they are fastened properly, all we need to do is to add these items to our checklist. Checklists are especially useful as they direct the nurse's attention to specific aspects of a patient's behaviour, previously selected as those areas where problems are particularly likely to arise. However they can become lengthy and cumbersome to use if care is not taken in selecting the right items for the checklist.

Counting, timing and checking require the nurse to observe and measure a particular behaviour at a specific time. The information about a patient gained by using these methods is therefore objective and contrasts in this respect with the information obtained by rating a behaviour.

Rating

Ratings are essentially judgements or opinions on a particular aspect of a patient's behaviour and thus always involve a subjective element. For this reason alone they are less reliable or stable than the other methods discussed but they can provide information which is often very useful in practice.

(a) A numerical scale

How well does the patient work?

1 Works unprompted
2 Needs occasional help
3 Needs supervision
4 Does not work without continuous supervision
5 Refuses to work

(b) A bipolar scale

How lengthy is patient's response to a question?

| Very lengthy response (Verbal diarrhoea) | Elaborate and lengthy response | Normal response | Very short yes/no answer | No answer (mute) |

(c) A unipolar scale

How bizarre is the patient's speech?

| Speech extremely bizarre | Speech frequently bizarre | Speech contains some bizarre ideas | Content of speech normal |

Fig. 3. Three types of rating scale.

They can be used to measure behaviour which is difficult to measure by any of the three methods already described such as those referring to the quality of a patient's performance. Consequently we can go some way to answering questions like 'How sociable is he?' and 'How co-operative is he with other people?'

In most rating scales the items consist of a question, and the observer answers by selecting the most appropriate answer from those provided, or by marking off on a line. *Fig.* 3 shows three scales: (a) a numerical scale, where the rater ticks the appropriate answer; and (b) and (c) where the rater marks the line at the point which he feels best describes the patient.

A bipolar scale has two poles or extremes and 'normal' lies in the middle, whereas on a unipolar scale there is only one pole or extreme—in the example given, it is not possible to be extremely unbizarre, so here 'normal' behaviour would be at the right-hand side of the scale.

Rating scales are useful in practice because they can save time in assessing a patient's behaviour. For example, a patient's behaviour over a period of time such as a week, leaves some impression on the rater, who can summarize this as a point on a scale, whereas measuring the behaviour with objective methods would require time spent each day in collecting data on the behaviour. However the rater's impression is made up of a haphazard composite of observations as it is not possible for him to see the patient in all situations and at all times during the week.

Whatever the problem behaviour we are attempting to measure, we should always try to use the most appropriate method which gives accurate results and does not take a large proportion of time to complete. Methods of measuring are not confined to these four presented for there may be others more relevant to a specific behaviour. Weighing for example is a particularly useful technique with problems of obesity, failure to eat meals and the wearing of an excessive number of clothes.

Most behaviours can be measured by using a single method, but two or more methods can be combined where different aspects of a behaviour are required. For example, where a patient has frequent outbursts of screaming and these persist for lengthy periods of time, we may want to measure both the total number of outbursts and the length of time of each screaming outburst.

RECORDING BEHAVIOUR

Carefully measured observations are of little value unless they are recorded in a way that enables them to be communicated. Brief written records are easy to understand at the moment they are made but become less easy to comprehend at later times. How often do we jot down a note and on discovering it a number of weeks later, are unable to understand it?

In order that our measurements can be of use, we generally enter them on a chart of some kind, the design of the chart being related to the type of measure used. All charts have a number of similar properties and certain precautions need to be taken when filling them in. These can be appropriately summarized under the following headings:

C — comprehend instructions
H — have events recorded immediately
A — awareness of errors
R — record clearly
T — take consistent measures
S — supply patients with information

Comprehend instructions

Even before observing a behaviour there are a few entries to be made and instructions to understand. A chart should always have spaces for the details of the patient's name and date to be inserted, and often spaces for

Name _____   Behaviour: Pacing

Pacing—walking in a way that covers
      the same ground for 3 out of 5
      minutes' observation
Observe every 1½ hours for 5 minutes
Time how long he paces in that
time and mark chart accordingly

KEY

Do not prompt patient not
to pace at any time

   ✓   Pacing (3 out of 5 minutes)

   X   Not pacing (less than 3 out
         of 5 minutes)

N/A Not applicable

Week Commencing_____	Mon	Tue	Wed	Thur	Fri	Sat	Sun	TOTAL
8·00 a.m.								
9·30 a.m.								
11·00 a.m.								
12·30								

Fig. 4. Chart designed to measure the behaviour of an individual patient.

the rater's name, and patient's ward. *Fig.* 4 shows a sample chart. The instructions include *what* exactly the behaviour is we are measuring. The definition of a behaviour will vary for each individual and his particular problem. Defining pacing, for example, as 'Walking without aim' is inadequate because of its subjectivity. How does the observer know if the patient has an aim? In *Fig.* 4, the definition of pacing for this particular patient was made as 'Walking in a way that covers the same ground for three out of five minutes observation'.

Defining a behaviour makes for more consistent ratings because all raters can then use the same criterion to discriminate between what is accepted and what is not. Whereas we would all have differing opinions as to what constitutes pacing, agreeing on a definition and writing this on the chart or in a ward manual helps everyone to work to the same rules.

In the example above, observers can only judge the patient to be pacing when the two criteria in the definition are fulfilled. The patient may walk around for 3 out of 5 minutes if he is sweeping the dining-room, for example, but he is not pacing unless he does so by repeatedly covering the same circuit. Alternatively, he could cover the same ground if he went from the sitting-room to his own room to collect some item and then returned because he had forgotten something, but this is also not classed as pacing unless he repeatedly does this for 3 out of 5 minutes.

Instructions as to *how* the measurements should be taken are also provided, whether it be counting, timing, checking or whatever. With rating scales, instructions in how to use the scales are often provided in some detail—such examples include: 'Answer each question by putting a tick in the box which you think best represents the patient as he has been during the last week', or 'Put a mark through the line at the point which you think best represents the patient's behaviour'.

Details of *when* to measure are also provided. Times may be fixed at once a day as in checking whether a patient is up at 7·15 a.m., or many times a day, where checks are made at meal times to see if the patient comes without being prompted. Times may be specified as in time sampling—for example, observing a patient for 5 minutes on every hour; or unspecified so that records are made when the behaviour occurs such as when the patient absconds. Measurement may also be made at the same time each day as checking every two hours to see if a patient is wearing his dentures; or at randomly planned times so one day an appearance check is made at 9·00 a.m. and the following day at 11·30 a.m.

A *key* shows which symbols to use to indicate various possibilities. These are often in the form of ticks and crosses, but with charts involving some kind of rating such symbols are not so relevant. A particularly useful method for measuring how much prompting patients needed during various tasks such as work, attending occupational therapy, arising and taking medication, was to involve a numbering system. 0 if the patient performed the task without any prompt, 1 if he required a prompt and 2 if he required a number of prompts or failed to do it altogether (*see Fig. 12 p. 132*). Keys should also indicate how the chart should be marked on the occasions where the behaviour cannot be observed. N/A for not applicable or N/O for not observed are useful symbols to use.

Charts frequently contain further instructions. They may refer to not prompting the patient, or relate to the reinforcing of a response such as 'Reward every third consecutive desirable response' or 'Reinforce every correct response with five tokens'.

Have events recorded immediately

If we fail to record events immediately, the details of the observation begin to fade from memory. Consequently a delayed record is no longer likely to be accurate. Alternatively, we may even forget to record it altogether! Sometimes it is possible to delay recording an event so remaining unobtrusive while observing the patient. We may be able to observe the *effects* of a behaviour rather than the behaviour itself. Thus if we wanted to know how well a patient washes the dishes, we can observe how clean they are afterwards, or if we wanted to know how well he makes his bed, we can check his bed later on, after he has done it. Since the behaviour of a patient changes the environment, we can in effect measure the patient's behaviour by measuring the environment.

This means the patient does not have to have someone standing over him all the time, with the anxiety that might arise. On the other hand we are then measuring the product, and not the process of washing pots or making the bed, but in many practical situations this does not matter.

Awareness of errors

If two people are asked to measure the height of a friend to the nearest one-thirty-secondth of an inch, they would probably disagree. Obviously the person's height has not changed so the error must come from the observer, and from variations in the observation situation. If simple physical measurements like this can lead to error, psychological measurements must also be prone to such error. The major components creating bias in psychological measures are the Halo effect and the Leniency error.

The *Halo effect* is the effect produced by the rater's general impression of the person he is rating. For example, if the first impression made by the patient is good, we will tend to rate him high on all characteristics. Conversely, if we see him as an 'awkward' patient, then all items relating to that patient will tend to be rated as 'bad'.

The *Leniency error* describes the tendency of raters to systematically rate all patients in a certain way. Some raters tend to be 'kind' to patients and systematically rate all patients as better than they 'really' are. A few raters may show the opposite effect, and being 'hard' on the patients makes them all seem worse. Guildford has classed both the constant tendency to rate too high or too low as leniency errors, but makes the point that the latter of the two tendencies is one of negative leniency.

Because ratings of a behaviour require more subjective judgements than counting, timing or checking a behaviour, they are obviously more prone to bias. By becoming aware that such errors exist, we can make a conscious effort to reduce them, so obtaining measurements which bear a closer resemblance to the patient's actual behaviour. One particularly useful method to remember when rating is to concentrate on the *behaviour* under observation, not the person doing it.

(a) <u>On a counting chart</u>

e.g. number of occurrences of head-banging.

Correction

	Mon.	Tue.
8·00	4̶4̶	6
9·00	1	0
10·00		2
11·00	4	2

Entry altered — Erase; use different colour

No entry because patient not on ward to be observed — Mark with 'not seen' or N/O.

(b) <u>On a checking chart</u>

	Mon.
Hair neat	✓
Tie on	/
Face clean	✓
Shirt buttoned	✓
Dentures worn	
Trousers clean	X
Socks on	✓
Shoes on	✗

Incorrect symbol: dash easily mistaken for tick — Refer to key: use X when item not present

No entry because not applicable: pt. has his own teeth — Refer to key: N/A used to refer to not applicable

Entry altered: tick changed to cross — Erase; use different colour

(c) <u>On a rating chart</u>

e.g. How much did the patient speak?

1. Mute

2. Monosyllable responses

3. Spoke in short sentences

✓ — — — — — — — — — — — — Behaviour judged to be between two items — Read instructions carefully — — — Ringing the number as an alternative method

4. Sentences generally short

5. As talkative as normal person

Fig. 5. Common errors in recording.

Record clearly

In charting observations, a variety of errors often occur which make the ratings difficult, often impossible to use. *Fig.* 5 illustrates some common errors.

They tend to arise through:
1. Entries being altered
2. Using symbols incorrectly
3. Not reading instructions clearly
4. Failing to make an entry

These can usually be remedied if a little time is taken in carefully reading the instructions, familiarizing ourselves with the key, clearly marking in entries and checking through to see all the items have been done. If, on checking, it becomes apparent that an entry has failed to be made, it is better to indicate this in some way, perhaps by stating 'not observed', rather than leaving it blank, but even leaving it blank is better than guessing at it!

Take consistent measures

Different people, seeing the same behaviour, may judge it differently, and the same person seeing the same behaviour at different times can also rate it differently. Such inconsistencies arise because of various reasons, the most common being:

1. Where the assessment situation is not standardized. Checking the cleanliness of a patient's face may produce a different result before and after a meal, especially if his eating habits are not good. Consistency can be increased by choosing standard times and places for measuring behaviour. However, this may not be appropriate, for some patients will learn to perform a behaviour only at the time of checking. For example, a patient may regularly have his dentures in when checked, but take them out immediately afterwards. In such cases a predetermined random check gives a more unbiased measure of his behaviour.

2. Where raters observe from different positions. Two people observing a patient from different angles see different things, and consequently a behaviour may be noticed by one and not by the other.

3. Where raters are not interested. Observers who do not understand what the recordings are for, and the use that will be made of them, are not motivated to fill charts in correctly.

4. Where raters have not agreed on a criterion of judgement. Two nurses may, for example, differ in their opinion as to whether they consider a patient's hair is tidy or not. Disagreement between raters should not be taken as a sign that one person is right and the other wrong, but should be the basis of discussion to agree on a criterion.

Supply patients with information

Often the patient himself is in the best position to record his own behaviour, and benefit from his involvement as assessor. Such instances include:

1. Where the nurse cannot record the behaviour. Patients with auditory hallucinations have filled in their own checklist on the presence or absence of hallucinations. This self-recording method has often produced a decrease in their hallucinations.

2. Where the patient may benefit from the additional feedback provided and consequent involvement and participation in the programme. By recording his own behaviour the patient becomes more aware of how he is doing. With one incontinent patient, the nurse checked his behaviour each morning and encouraged him to fill in the chart by the side of his bed, with a tick when he was 'dry' and a cross on the mornings he was 'wet'.

3. Where targets can be entered on a chart so patients can see their progress towards a goal. The target for one patient was to come for his meals six out of eight times without being prompted to earn an extra privilege. By entering this target on a self-recording chart he could see his own progress and was given a further incentive to reach his target.

When such self-recording techniques are used, the method of marking the chart may need to be modified. For one patient ticks and crosses proved to be of little value, but red stars for good performances produced more interest in recording and led to an improvement in his behaviour.

PRESENTATION OF RECORDINGS

Charts which are used to record initial observations are only of short-term value, since they usually can only carry information for a week or two's observations. However, the original chart is still of value. It contains data from events in the immediate past, which may be of use to the nurse at that present moment. Where the nurse needs to reinforce not every response but every third response, for example, then she can immediately refer to the patient's previous responses and work out at which point to reinforce.

Charts also enable information to be transferred from one nurse to another. Each can find out, for example, how many days a patient has gone without wetting his bed, or what time he got up in the morning. By the sharing of this objective information staff become more consistent in their approach and consequently patients are not confused by different members of staff doing different things.

The act of filling in a chart may help the nurse to direct her attention to a patient's problem which might otherwise have gone unnoticed. For example, if it is obvious that a patient's face is dirty when doing a hygiene check, we might well start to think about how to encourage him to keep it clean.

The mass of information contained on a chart can be simplified by using a graph. Graphs have the ability to store information over a much

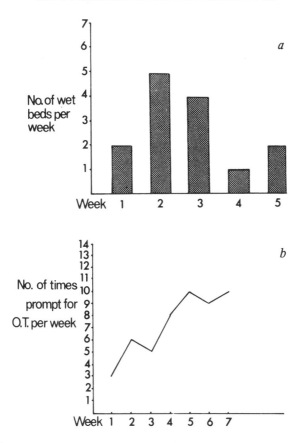

Fig. 6. Types of graphs. *a,* Bar graph ('histogram'), showing frequency of incontinence. *b,* Line graph, showing number of times that patient is on time for O.T.

longer period of time and can be interpreted easily by eye. *Fig.* 6 shows the two main kinds of graph:

Bar graphs (or histograms) are made up of a series of vertical bars, the heights of which represent the extent to which the behaviour has been performed during each observation period.

Line graphs are a series of points connected with each other by a line, each point representing a successive measurement. The distance of the point from the bottom horizontal line of the graph represents the level of behaviour. Both these examples show *raw* scores; that is, the actual number of occurrences is recorded. However, where the number of observations are not constant from week to week a raw score cannot be

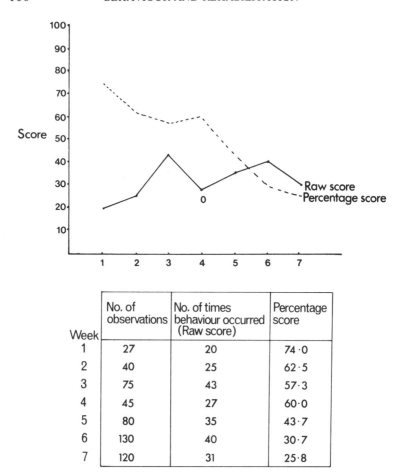

Week	No. of observations	No. of times behaviour occurred (Raw score)	Percentage score
1	27	20	74·0
2	40	25	62·5
3	75	43	57·3
4	45	27	60·0
5	80	35	43·7
6	130	40	30·7
7	120	31	25·8

Fig. 7. Difference in graphs plotted from the raw score and percentage score, where the number of observations vary.

used. For example, in *Fig.* 6b a number of the possible 14 observations may be missed one week because the patient spends a day at home, or has to go for treatment to another department. Where the number of observations are not constant from week to week, the raw scores have to be corrected so they are comparable. This can be done by using the following formula which gives a percentage score:

$$\frac{\text{No. of events observed}}{\text{No. of observations}} \times 100$$

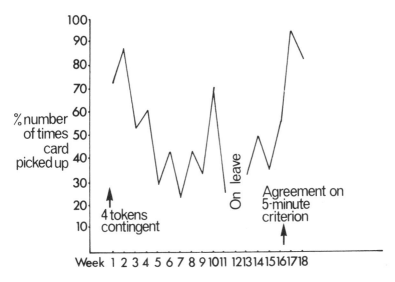

Fig. 8. Inconsistent reinforcement by different shifts producing weekly alteration in response.

Thus if in graph 6 b, the patient was not on the ward for two sessions of O.T. during the week, the maximum number of possible observations would be 12. Now if we consider that he is prompt on nine of these occasions, his percentage score would be:

$$\frac{9}{12} \times 100 = 75\%$$

Percentage scores can be graphed in the same way as raw scores but they must not be added or averaged as the scores will become meaningless.

If the raw scores fail to be corrected where the number of observations are not constant, a false picture can be produced. *Fig.* 7 shows there to be no overall change in behaviour when raw scores are plotted, but when the scores are corrected to take into account the different number of observations, the true picture emerges—the plotted percentage scores show occurrences of the behaviour gradually decrease.

Graphs provide information which helps to build up a history of the patient's behaviour patterns, so forming a permanent record which we can refer to at any later date. We can find out for instance by how much a patient's behaviour has improved, what produced the change and how long it took, which may be of use in designing further treatment programmes. We can also discover whether present treatment is effective or not, and consequently change it to benefit the patient.

Where the patient's responses are plotted on a graph and show improvement in behaviour, it can be reinforcing for the nurse. We are able to see a visual record of the patient's behaviour resulting from a treatment which we have participated in.

Graphs may also indicate why a patient may not be responding to treatment. One patient was rewarded with tokens every time she picked up her job card (which indicated the ward jobs she was to do), in an effort to increase her initiative. Her response is shown in *Fig.* 8. The graph suggests a weekly alteration in the patient's behaviour. Inspection of this showed it to be coincidental with the number of possible reinforcing events each shift was responsible for (twice on a morning and once on an afternoon shift) which also alternated each week. This suggested different shifts were not being consistent in the way they carried out the programme—in fact, one shift had allowed her 5 minutes to pick up the card after a meal, and the other shift about 2 minutes. Agreeing on a specific time led to an immediate improvement in behaviour.

Chapter 10

WHAT'S THE PROBLEM?

The number and variety of behavioural problem patients on long-stay wards possess are vast. Some problems are difficult to detect unless we stand back and analyse what is going on. Others are more easily observed especially if the patient has just started behaving in this way. In communicating these observations to others concerned with the patient's welfare it is easy to give statements like, 'Mr Jones has no idea how to set the table', 'Arthur never wears his dentures', 'Harry seems depressed today', 'Fred's a messy eater', and 'Jill has been pacing all morning'. Statements like these, however, serve very little purpose for they are both *interpretative* and probably *exaggerated.*

By interpretative we mean that instead of describing what the patient actually *does,* we make an interpretation of his behaviour. For example, the observer making statements such as those above inferred that because Harry was seen speaking slowly, in the same tone, and stopped several times to sob, he was depressed. Another observer might have inferred something quite different. Similarly what does messy eating mean? The term 'messy eating' covers a host of odd behaviours and to label Fred's behaviour as such tells us nothing about his specific eating problems. We need to know whether Fred is messy because he eats with his hands, because he spills food down his shirt or because he spits his food out. In addition, to say Mr Jones has 'no idea' how to set the table involves a dubious assumption. He may very well have some idea how to set the table, but fails to put the behaviour into action for one of a number of reasons.

By exaggerated statements we mean the tendency to attribute a patient with some behaviour or lack of some behaviour because he has been observed behaving in such a way on a few occasions. Has Jill really been pacing *all* morning—during the times she spent washing, dressing, eating breakfast, taking medication and through coffee breaks? Similarly is it true to say that Arthur *never* ever wears his dentures—not even at meal times?

Behaviour problems usually first come to notice in one of two ways:
1. Through the patient's inability to perform adequately during part of the regular routine. He may, for example, be unable to arise on a morning without persistent prompting, having messy eating habits at the meal table, or be unable to concentrate on his basket work at a session of occupational therapy.
2. The behaviour may become conspicuous independently of the routine, so speech problems, incontinence and destructive behaviour may be detected for example. With the discovery of a problem, the first stage is to describe it accurately.

DESCRIBING BEHAVIOUR

Behaviour is any action of a person which can be observed, and therefore if a person's behaviour is unusual or abnormal enough to be a problem, it should be specified as a set of actions. Intent should never be attributed to a person's behaviour but the behaviour just described in specific concrete and observable terms.

Should a patient throw his work on the floor, thump the table, shout a couple of obscenities and go and kick the door, it helps little if we say he is 'aggressive'. This would be an inference from his behaviour. Aggressive behaviour can be interpreted differently by a selection of individuals. Some may think of aggression as throwing and breaking objects, others as hitting another person, neither of which the patient did. Everyone concerned with the patient's treatment should know exactly what the problem is, and this can only be achieved if the behaviour is objectively observed and reliably described. When the problem is described accurately it can readily be identified by a number of different people.

In the behavioural approach, we observe behaviour without making assumptions and inferences about 'internal' hidden motivations. Hence the statement 'Joe talks about staff members stealing his money and about not being paid the wage he deserves at occupational therapy' is a more behaviourally descriptive statement of the patient's behaviour, than saying 'Joe has delusions of persecution'. Further examples of the difference between interpretative and behavioural descriptions may be those shown in *Table* 1.

Abnormal behaviour among chronic patients can be described either in terms of: (1) a *handicap* to the patient—where behaviour is present it is performed inappropriately; or (2) a *deficiency* in the patient's behavioural repertoire.

Behavioural handicaps are those behaviours which because of their extreme form (e.g. throwing and breaking objects, head banging) or their increased frequency (e.g. continually talking to self, excessive pacing,

Table 1. Interpretative and behavioural descriptions

Interpretative description (inference or interpretation)	Behavioural description
1. He has lost his confidence	He did no work for an hour at occupational therapy, but sat gazing out of the window and did not talk to anyone.
2. He seems hostile	He smashed an empty plate on the floor during dinner.
3. He was hallucinating	He sat in a corner and talked to himself.

and obsessively checking a door is locked) restrict the patient's adaptation to his environment. They handicap his existence in a social environment, because of their 'embarrassing' quality.

Behavioural deficiencies, on the other hand, refer to those behaviours expected of a patient but which he fails to perform. Such deficits can occur as a result of lack of practice. So we may observe a patient with untidy hair, and notice that on occasions such as the weekly social, when he requires to be tidy, it is the nurse who combs his hair. We might say the behaviour of combing hair has been 'lost' to the patient through lack of opportunity and practice. Quite a number of behavioural deficiencies are the result of such institutionalization. Alternatively, a patient may be deficient in some aspect of his behavioural repertoire through never having learnt the skill, either because of non-training as with the mentally handicapped, or because of the patient's social and cultural background.

This distinction between behaviours described as handicaps and deficiencies becomes important when treatment of the problem is considered. Handicaps need to be reduced and replaced with positive adaptive behaviour whereas deficient behaviour is overcome through the training of specific skills.

Approaching the description of behavioural handicaps and deficiencies may be quite different. With handicaps, a description may be quite simple (e.g. 'He is incontinent of urine') but often it is more complex than this. An objective description of the patient's behaviour will often reveal a number of 'undesirable behaviours' which make up the handicap. For example, the 'aggressive' patient's behaviour discussed earlier, consisted of four inappropriate behaviours; throwing dinner on the floor, thumping the table, shouting obscenities and kicking the door. Therefore, here we have four behaviours, not one, with which to deal. Sometimes the inappropriate behaviour may be a *component* of a behaviour. Walking, for example, consists of a number of components, any or all of which may be inappropriate and give walking an 'odd' appearance. A patient may shuffle instead of stride (one component), walk with arms folded instead of down by the side (second component) and/or walk with arched instead of straight back (a third component).

With behavioural deficiencies it is often helpful to describe the behaviour in terms of how it fails to approach normality. This may be achieved through a series of questions:

1. *Does he perform the behaviour?*
   Yes   No—e.g. he does not speak; he fails to dress himself.

2. *Does he do it well?*
   Yes   No—e.g. he may dress himself, but do so badly giving a poor appearance; he may make his bed but fail to make an adequate job of it.

3. *Does he do it without a nurse prompting him?*
   Yes   No—e.g. he may have the ability to get out of bed on a morning or be able to come for his meal but require a number of prompts to perform the behaviour. It is not spontaneous behaviour.

4. *Does he do it at the appropriate time?*
   Yes   No—e.g. he may go to bed in the afternoon; he washes his hair when dinner is being served.

5. *Does he do it at the appropriate place?*
   Yes   No—e.g. lying on the floor rather than the bed; urinating down the stairs rather than in the toilet.

6. *Does he do it within a reasonable time limit?*
   Yes   No—e.g. he takes 3 hours to mop the bathroom; he waits until everyone finishes their meal before he starts.

7. *Does he maintain the behaviour?*
   Yes   No—e.g. his appearance soon becomes dirty and untidy.

8. *In what other respects is his behaviour undesirable?*

DEFINING BEHAVIOUR

Once a behaviour has been described it requires definition. This has been discussed in relation to measuring, and involves stating for each individual the behaviour in such objective terms that any observer seeing the behaviour can judge it in similar ways and record it accurately.

Behaviour handicaps

With behavioural handicaps the definition usually focuses upon the problem behaviour in question. If hoarding for one patient consists of the accumulation of used and irrelevant items in a handbag (a description), then for this patient the definition of hoarding may go something like 'the accumulation of empty cigarette or match boxes in the handbag'. Some may think this rather strict, stressing that 'normally' people often carry the odd empty box about until they have a chance to empty their bag. The definition may then be altered to: 'the accumulation of more than one empty cigarette or match box in the handbag'.

Again, it might become apparent that some of the boxes are not empty, but contain dead matches or cigarette ends. What should we do about this? Do we class such boxes as not hoarded because they are not empty or do we alter the definition further to include such occurrences. Hoarding might then be defined for this person as 'the accumulation of more than one cigarette packet or match box which does not contain appropriate items, in the handbag'. We could go further to consider what to do in the event of other types of empty box being in the handbag, or of empty match boxes hoarded on the person. These problems have to be discussed when everyone concerned with the treatment is present, and a consensus of opinion reached, and adhered to. The definition of each problem for each individual will accordingly differ quite markedly, even if the problem behaviour for two individuals can be loosely classed under the one heading such as 'hoarding'.

A definition often involves outlining a number of criteria, all of which have to be fulfilled before a behaviour can be said to be similar to the one under investigation. With head-rubbing for example there may be three criteria:

1. That any part of either or both hands must be touching any part of the head above the neck.
2. That there must be a rubbing movement, to and fro.
3. That this must persist continuously for 5 seconds or more.

This definition then would exclude any behaviour from being called head rubbing if it did not fulfil all three criteria. A still hand on the head for 5 seconds or over, or a rubbing with the hand on the head for less than 5 seconds would, by this definition, not be called head-rubbing.

Behavioural deficiencies

With behavioural deficiencies, rather than define the patient's behaviour it is frequently more practical to define the behaviour expected of him. For example, it would be difficult to define 'a lack of arising behaviour' but not so hard to define the expected or 'normal' arising behaviour. It may be defined for one individual as 'out of bed before 7·10 a.m. with only one prompt by nurse' and from this we can measure how deficient the patient's behaviour is, for every morning on which he fails to fulfil the criteria would be charted as a failure to respond.

Similarly the appearance of a patient can be measured by using a checklist composed of various items ranging from 'hair neat' through 'shirt on' to 'shoes fastened'. Each item requires a definition so anyone using the checklist would be consistent in their judgement of what 'hair neat', 'shirt on' and so forth meant. For example, the criteria needed to be fulfilled for a patient to be considered as having his 'shirt on' appropriately may be that he has it on the right way round, that he has his arms down both sleeves, that the front is buttoned and that he has it tucked into the top of his trousers.

BASELINE

A baseline is a measure of the extent of a problem—a record of the patient's behaviour before the introduction of any treatment. After the behavioural problem has been defined we can set about designing a suitable baseline chart, the form of which will depend like any other, upon precisely what is being measured. We require baseline measures for two reasons:

1. To discover the full range of problems, and to pinpoint the most important. For example, carrying out a baseline check on the appearance of a patient might reveal only one or two of the items are consistently rated as performed poorly whilst performance on all other items is adequate. Analysis of the results may thus reveal important implications for treatment. In this case, that treatment should be focused on the one or two particular items, rather than an attempt made to treat 'appearance' in a global fashion.

2. To judge the effectiveness of any treatment which we decide to carry out with the patient. Any change from the baseline level of behaviour indicates how effective, or ineffective, that treatment has been in changing behaviour.

The duration of a baseline depends both upon the rate at which observations are made, and upon the reliability of these observations. The length of a baseline is related to the frequency with which the behaviour in question occurs. For example, 'talking to self' or 'mannerisms' can be checked more frequently than 'washing hair' or 'goes to hospital social'. Therefore, depending upon the frequency of behaviour, an accurate baseline may accordingly last a week or two, or in some cases even a month or two months.

In considering reliability of observations, we sometimes find measurements of behaviour vary quite markedly from week to week for no apparent reason. Rather than take an average from these recordings, it is better to attempt to discover why the discrepancies have occurred. They may be due, for example, to different recording techniques of staff, or to differences in behaviour at different times of the day. If and when the reason for such discrepancies is established it may be necessary to carry out further baseline measures to correct earlier errors.

A problem frequently encountered in carrying out baseline observations is that treatment may effectively begin unwittingly. Whenever a patient observes someone checking his behaviour he may pick up prompts or cues and act on these by altering his behaviour. Treatment can then be said to have begun. It is then virtually impossible to obtain a reliable estimate of how bad the patient's behaviour is. Behaviours such as hoarding, which necessarily make the patient aware of the assessment procedure, are vulnerable to this sort of effect during baseline recordings. To avoid such bias or error in baseline measures, we should attempt to keep the patient unaware he is being measured. During baselines, in contrast to treatment, the patient should ideally be ignorant of our presence and motive. This is sometimes difficult to achieve but errors introduced by the observer can be reduced by:

(*a*) Checking the *results* of a behaviour rather than the behaviour itself. For example, we may count the number of burn holes a patient makes in her dress at a time she is not wearing it, rather than observe the actual behaviour of dress burning.

(*b*) Behaving in a way which is not obviously an assessment procedure. For example, if we are sitting with a group of patients observing their interactions we may decide to use the squares of a crossword puzzle to mark off when particular interactions we are interested in occur. The patient is thus given the impression we are reading. Similarly we may ask a patient to 'Give us a smile' when we need to discover if he is wearing his dentures.

There are two other events which we might be interested to discover during the baseline, and which may lend help in designing a treatment for the patient's problem. These are the *antecedents* (under what conditions does the behaviour generally occur) and the *consequences* (what usually happens when the patient performs the undesirable behaviour).

Let us consider a behaviour problem such as outbursts of shouting. After defining the behaviour we would need to take a baseline measure of how often it occurred, but in addition it might be useful to chart the antecedents of each outburst. For example, we might make a note of the situation and in whose presence the behaviour occurred. When analysing this information it may become clear the patient shouts and curses more during sessions of group activities than at other times, or only in the presence of one particular person. We may then require to know what it is about such a situation that causes the patient to shout and curse. When we are able to identify the antecedents, we may be able to modify the environment in such a way that the behaviour is no longer 'triggered'. Particular examples of this are given in Chapter 15.

The consequences of a behaviour are also important to document, and the best way of doing this is to note exactly what happens when the behaviour occurs. When a patient starts shouting, do the nurses come running to find out what is wrong, is the patient taken out from a group activity or is he given a cigarette to calm him down? This is important to know for it may provide a clue as to what the most appropriate treatment should be.

Analysis of baseline data may reveal interesting information which is independent of the particular behaviour being measured. For example, *Fig.* 9 shows an example of inconsistent rating. On weeks 2 and 4 the patient, according to the observer, failed to get up in the morning every time, whereas on weeks 1 and 3 he arose approximately half of the time.

Week Number
1   2   3   4

	1	2	3	4	
Sun	✓	x	x	x	KEY:
Mon	✓	x	x	x	✓ Out of bed by 7·10
Tue	x	x	x	x	x Still in bed at 7·10
Wed	✓	x	✓	x	N/O Not observed
Thur	x	x	✓	x	
Fri	✓	x	x	x	
Sat	✓	x	✓	x	
TOTAL	5	0	3	0	

Fig. 9. A baseline chart recording the occurrence of arising behaviour.

Such a pattern may indicate a different recording procedure was being carried out on alternative weeks, which would coincide with shift changes and should prompt further investigation into the discrepancy between shifts. One shift may, for example, have prompted the patient a number of times between 7·00 and 7·10 a.m. whilst the other shift may have given just one call and a check at 7·10. Here, in order to obtain a reliable baseline, we need to ensure staff are being consistent in their approach and recording of the patient's behaviour.

Let us consider a patient persistently leaving the ward without permission. *Fig.* 10 shows a chart for one week designed to discover the amount that a patient was absent without leave (A.W.O.L.). Suppose we took this baseline for 4 weeks and discovered an almost identical pattern occurred each time. Two things would become clear:

(*a*) The patient leaves the ward between 12·30 and 2·00 p.m., the time during which ward staff meetings are also held. Thus he leaves when he is less likely to be missed and once he has left he stays out all afternoon.

	Sun	Mon	Tue	Wed	Thur	Fri	Sat
8 · 30	✓	✓	✓	✓	✓	✓	✓
9 · 30	✓	✓	✓	✓	✓	✓	✓
10 · 30	✓	✓	✓	✓	✓	✓	✓
11 · 30	✓	✓	N/O	✓	✓	✓	✓
12 · 30	✓	✓	✓	✓	✓	✓	✓
2 · 00	✓	x	✓	✓	✓	x	✓
3 · 00	✓	x	✓	✓	✓	x	✓
4 · 00	✓	x	✓	✓	✓	x	N/O
5 · 00	✓	x	✓	✓	✓	x	N/O
6 · 00	✓	x	✓	✓	✓	x	✓
TOTAL A.W.O.L	0	5	0	0	0	5	0

KEY: ✓ Patient is on ward

     x Patient is absent from ward

     N/O Not observed

Fig. 10. A baseline chart recording A.W.O.L. for one patient.

(*b*) He leaves the ward only and always on Mondays and Fridays. If we investigate the case a little deeper we might try to discover where in fact he goes when he leaves the ward. In this case it soon becomes apparent because his mother rings the ward to inform the staff that he is at her house. On looking through the visitors' book we find, however, that his mother visits him regularly. Discussion with the mother and patient finally pin-points the problem. He goes home when he has run out of money. As he is given his money on Saturdays and Wednesdays it becomes clear that his difficulties lie in the area of budgeting—he is spent out by Monday and Friday. This demonstrates the importance of finding and treating the main problem—in this case not one of leaving the ward but one of budgeting.

Where a patient has a number of behaviour problems, consideration should be given to the problem of which behaviour to treat first. This involves:

The seriousness of the problem. Smearing and eating faeces would therefore be considered a major problem and be amongst the first treated. Domestic and social skill training must wait with such a patient until he has learned the more basic self-care behaviours. In general, self-care or self-help skills should be the first behaviours taught where these are lacking.

The feasibility in terms of the patient's routine activities. Treatment to increase a patient's denture wearing, for example, can be held up if he is never up in time for his breakfast. Arising on time would therefore be considered a problem deserving treatment before denture wearing.

When a baseline confirms a behaviour problem does exist, before initiating treatment it is worth considering whether there is a physical reason for the behaviour? Answering this may involve us in considering such diverse causes as an infection which may be causing incontinence, ill-fitting dentures which are not worn because they hurt the patient, or excessive night sedation resulting in a lack of arising on time.

SECTION IV
TREATMENT

Chapter 11

POSITIVE REINFORCERS

A positive reinforcer, as we have already discussed, is *anything* which increases the frequency or improves the quality of a behaviour it follows. Treatment involves the identification and utilization of reinforcers. It is important to discover what is reinforcing for each individual, if treatment is going to be maximally effective. Basically, there are four types of reinforcer:

1. Social reinforcers
2. Material reinforcers
3. Privileges
4. Tokens

1. SOCIAL REINFORCERS

These include the giving of attention and verbal or non-verbal approval. They were discussed at some length in the discussion of nurse–patient interaction and have the advantage of being reinforcing for most patients. Because they occur naturally and are always available to the person who is reinforcing, they are very practical and can be given immediately desirable behaviour occurs. Some problems in using social reinforcers in treatment are: (a) they are difficult to record; (b) the patient can become too dependent on approval; and (c) they are difficult to control. We have seen how nurses may pay attention to undesirable behaviour. One nurse behaving in such a way can destroy a whole team's effort, for she will maintain the inappropriate behaviour even though the patient may behave appropriately to other members of staff. In addition, during individual sessions with a patient, a certain amount of attention is

119

available all the time by virtue of the nurse's presence, so there may be much unintentional reinforcement occurring. Even the act of rating a patient which is not usually regarded as reinforcing may in fact be so.

2. MATERIAL REINFORCERS

These refer to items immediately present, or tangible pleasurable things usually small enough to be given repeatedly. They include items of food, drinks, sweets, cigarettes and magazines, and are potentially very powerful reinforcers. With long-stay patients, cigarettes are often very strong reinforcers as indicated by the amount of time spent hunting for 'ends' when a whole cigarette is not available. However, the bigger the item, the less easy it is to apply contingently upon 'good' behaviour, both because it becomes impracticable and because the patient may become satiated. It is not practicable, for instance, to reinforce a patient's behaviour with a meal, if there is a time delay between the behaviour and when the meal occurs. It is also often unpractical for the nurse to carry the reinforcer around in her uniform so that she can be in a position to reinforce immediately, because of the size or weight of the reinforcers. Patients also become quickly satiated with a reinforcer if it is given in large quantities. For example, a patient given a bar of chocolate for uttering a word or two will quickly be in a position of not desiring any more chocolate, and so the reinforcer loses its value. When material reinforcers are used they should be given in 'bits'. Thus part of a meal, sips of a drink or squares of a bar of chocolate are more useful than giving the reinforcer as a whole, since they can be repeatedly given with little satiation.

3. PRIVILEGES

These are events not usually given for each instance of the behaviour, but for repeatedly successful performance. They include such events as coffee breaks, staying in bed in the morning, use of a particular favourite chair, a single room to sleep in, a trip down town and freedom from usual ward restrictions.

It is advisable not to deprive patients of items they are accustomed to having. Rather reinforcers that are not ordinarily available should be sought and added to the list of potential reinforcements.

4. TOKENS

A token is basically a symbol standing for some other reinforcer. Tokens are not reinforcing in themselves but become reinforcing because they are able to be exchanged for items the patient desires. Thus they are called *secondary* reinforcers because they gain reinforcing value by being associated with a stimulus that is reinforcing. Social and material reinforcers, in contrast, are *primary* reinforcers as their reinforcing value does not have to be learnt in the same way.

Real currency, 'money off' coupons and stamps given with goods at the supermarket are all tokens with which we are familiar, and which would be valueless if we were not able to exchange them for goods we require. The tokens used in patients' treatment programmes may include plastic discs, imitation toy money, points, punched cards or tickets, the actual form having little significance in itself. Its major importance is that when earned for appropriate behaviour the currency can always be honoured. A token only has value in the setting in which it is used, and so any tokens a patient earned on the ward, for example, can be spent only in this setting unless arrangements are made for the patient to spend them at the hospital shop or at other places such as a canteen.

Tokens are a useful way of reinforcing behaviour and have many advantages over other kinds of reinforcers:

(*a*) They are *easily recorded.* The amount of social and material reinforcer given to patients cannot be judged as easily as the amount of tokens given.

(*b*) The individual has a *choice* in how he wants to spend his tokens, and thus the item or event chosen has a greater chance of being reinforcing. Additionally, the same token reinforcer can be given to individuals who have different preferences in 'back-up' reinforcers. A 'back-up' reinforcer refers to the item or event the patient chooses to spend his tokens on.

(*c*) They can be *easily carried about* by staff in large quantities, usually being small enough to fit into the nurse's pocket.

(*d*) They are *tangible,* the patient having the tokens in his possession even when away from the situation in which he earned them.

(*e*) They are *durable,* in comparison to cigarettes and food which can easily be damaged by being carried about.

(*f*) There is *no satiation* because tokens can be used for anything the patient wishes to buy. Tokens, like money, are of equal value at any time whereas food, a material reinforcer, loses its value after a meal. We would not be motivated to work for food, having just finished off a feast, but we are likely to work for money regardless of how much we have in our possession.

(*g*) *Stealing* can be controlled either by keeping a check on the amount of tokens given or by using special tokens, perhaps of a different colour, for potential 'victims'.

(*h*) They can be given *continuously* during treatment. The treatment of a mute patient reinforced with boiled sweets for making any sound would be frequently held up whilst the patient finished the sweet. Tokens avoid this, allowing the patient to accumulate them throughout a session and exchange them later for items he wishes to purchase.

(*i*) They have an *educational* value. Some long-stay patients have forgotten how to count, and for many decimal coinage is something entirely foreign. Tokens in the form of plastic imitation money can be useful in addition to their reinforcing value in teaching patients to count, deal with money and how to save and bank.

(*j*) They *bridge the delay* between a desired response and a reinforcer. In this way many privileges and material reinforcers can be used, the patient earning tokens for appropriate behaviour which he then exchanges at a later time for 'back-up' items. One loud and aggressive female patient, for example, received tokens for being quiet throughout the day, and was then able to exchange these in the evening for a bag of make-up and entrance to the hospital social.

(*k*) The number of tokens given can bear a *simple quantitative relationship* to the amount considered necessary. In this way more difficult or less preferred ward tasks can be adjusted to be worth more tokens.

(*l*) They can be easily *controlled* in comparison to attention as a reinforcer, and can only be obtained for selected desirable behaviour.

(*m*) Using tokens involves a *two way process*—the giving of the reinforcer and the exchanging for the desired goods. This, in comparison to 'one way' primary reinforcers, produces increased encounters between nurse and patient and further increases the planned number of therapeutic interactions occurring.

Using tokens is not always the most effective way of reinforcing behaviour. Perhaps we should redress the balance and state some of the disadvantages of using tokens in treatment programmes:

(*a*) It can create extra administration, especially if a number of patients are on a token system, in assessing the amount each behaviour is worth, costing the various 'back-up' items, and keeping up to date recordings of what each patient has earned and spent.

(*b*) Giving tokens for some behaviours such as speech seems 'artificial'.

(*c*) Some patients, the very regressed, may have to learn first that tokens are of value, and learn not to throw them away or give them to other patients.

(*d*) There may be a long delay between earning the token and the presentation of the reinforcer, too long for some patients. However, this delay may be advantageous for other patients—those of a higher level—steering them away from living for the 'here and now' they may have grown used to and teaching them to save, budget and look forward to scheduled events.

(*e*) Staff who come to rely almost exclusively on token reinforcers may lose or fail to develop other and often more desirable means of reinforcing behaviour. We should never lose sight of the importance of social reinforcers in the development of patients' behaviour.

(*f*) A patient being reinforced with tokens may come to expect payment for appropriate behaviour and may refuse to behave appropriately without it. Where such situations arise, we need to reduce the tie or association between payment and behaviour so that the behaviour is executed spontaneously. Means to achieving this include techniques of planned token removal rather than sudden removal. These are discussed under the section on 'weaning'.

FINDING A REINFORCER

Before choosing reinforcers to use in a treatment programme, we have to discover to the best of our ability which will be most effective. This involves finding out what is reinforcing for each particular patient and can be achieved in various ways:

1. Asking the patient
2. Using a checklist
3. Utilizing requests and/or complaints
4. Observing the patient's behaviour
5. Reinforcer sampling

Asking the patient. This we would do automatically, although in practice it is not necessarily the best way of discovering reinforcers. Some patients may be mute or speak very little so fail to answer, others, the most withdrawn and institutionalized patients, often answer, 'Nothing', or give a very limited range of items such as, 'Cigs, that's all'. Alternatively some patients may say things they do not particularly want and are not prepared to 'earn' once the item is available. Thus, one patient said he liked salmon, but when a tin of it was made available to him at the ward shop he would not purchase it, preferring to spend his tokens on other things.

Despite these drawbacks it is always worth while initially asking patients what they like for it is the most natural and easiest way to discover potential reinforcers. Where patients ask for expensive items such as a tin of salmon, or a new dress, it is worth while asking them to leave a deposit of some kind (e. g. a number of tokens). This safeguards against accumulating items patients ask for but do not purchase.

Using a checklist. This is a list of items which can range from a host of edible products to social events and material objects as in *Fig.* 11. The list is read through with the patient and those items which he indicates he likes are checked off. Though certainly not exhaustive of all the possible reinforcers in the patient's environment a checklist does provide the patient with many ideas not immediately apparent to him.

However, there can sometimes be so many items on a checklist as to make it a laborious technique to use, since a lot of the items are

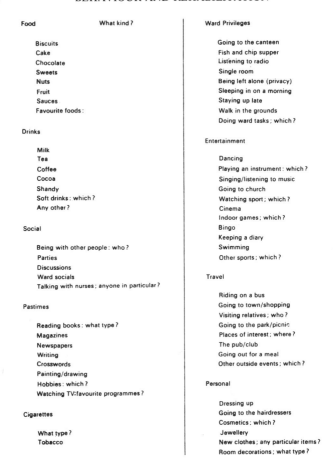

Fig. 11. Checklist for discovering potential reinforcers for female patients.

redundant. When completed we have a list of items the patient likes but no means to discriminate between them, so consequently no indication of which he prefers best amongst them, and the degree of preference is important in designing an effective treatment programme. Checklists, in addition, fail to overcome the problem of patients saying things they do not want. In fact it is probably made even easier for the patient to do so, since he only has to respond with a 'Yes' or 'No' to each item.

Utilizing patients' requests and/or complaints. This is a very useful and effective means of finding potential positive reinforcers, for if an institutionalized patient requests or complains about something, it is usually something he really wants, or wants rid of. However, this method is often overlooked as a means to finding a reinforcer. As an example of how this can be utilized, let us consider a patient who complained he was not being given enough medication. A typical response to this complaint might have been to see the doctor about more medication, comfort the patient by assuring him he was being given sufficient pills or even to ignore his complaints. However, this was viewed as an opportunity to develop the range of reinforcers for this patient. Placebo pills looking exactly like the patient's medication, but in fact containing no medication at all, were prescribed by the doctor. These were then used as part of a treatment programme, where the patient was able to purchase 'extra medication' with tokens he earned for behaving in a desirable fashion.

A problem with using this method in discovering potential reinforcers is that requests and/or complaints apart from ones concerning cigarettes, occur only infrequently, and hence may be thought of, or discovered only once treatment has begun.

Observe the patient's behaviour. One way of choosing an appropriate and effective reinforcer for a patient is simply to observe what he does when left to himself. This is based on *Premack's Principle,* which emphasizes that any behaviour which is preferred or frequently engaged in by a person can be used as a reinforcer for other less preferred or infrequent behaviours. In other words, whatever the patient spends a lot of time doing, can be used as a reinforcer, and so in this sense, there must always be potential reinforcers for a patient.

Ayllon and Azrin were the first to apply this principle to the treatment of long-stay patients. Patients worked at hospital jobs (less preferred or less frequent behaviours) to earn tokens which could then be exchanged for the chance to spend 30 minutes sitting in a favourite chair (highly preferred or high frequency behaviour). Other high-frequency behaviours common to long-stay patients, and which therefore may be potential reinforcers are watching TV, lying on a bed and, for some, talking to a nurse. 'Doing nothing' is a key reinforcer for many institutionalized patients, and it may be possible to utilize this. A patient earning tokens for his appearance may therefore be allowed to spend them on the privilege of opting out of certain activities on the ward.

The difficulty in using this technique to find potential reinforcers is that it involves taking a measurement on what the patient actually does, which usually lasts one to two weeks. However, this can often be taken whilst the baseline is being taken, so no time is lost. In practical terms it is sometimes difficult to use a reinforcer found by this method. Without special facilities or constant staff surveillance it is difficult to build reinforcers, like watching television, or sitting in a favourite chair, into a treatment programme.

Reinforcer sampling. Often a number of potential reinforcers will not be immediately apparent to long-stay patients, since through their stay in hospital they become used to the institutionalized style of life. Once patients are allowed to sample 'new' items and events these can become reinforcing. Thus if a patient is allowed to sample a single room, napkins on his meal table, a trip to the cinema, a fish-and-chip supper or shopping in town, these events achieve value as reinforcers if the patient expresses a desire to participate in them again. Such reinforcers can then be made contingent on appropriate behaviour.

However, long-stay patients may refuse to co-operate in sampling an event, their apathy overriding any mild curiosity they may have. In such circumstances a patient may be enticed into sampling an item or event by watching others participate in it. For example, in the dining area a patient may see others paying tokens to sit at a table which has tablecloths, napkins and a vase of flowers, or he may see other patients coming back from town with items they have purchased at the shops. This is exactly how a number of advertisements work—they direct our attention to someone using a particular product and the desirable consequences that follow from using it, and thus we become tempted to sample the product so that we may also obtain the desirable consequences.

EFFECTIVENESS OF A REINFORCER

There are a number of factors which determine how effective a reinforcer will be in changing behaviour. Some of these, such as the way it is given (e.g. immediately, sincerely, naturally) were discussed in Chapter 6, but there are many other factors.

One important aspect is the 'strength' of the reinforcer. Following Premack's Principle we see that for any patient there are a number of potential reinforcers but some will be more reinforcing for a patient than others. The 'strength' of a reinforcer can be judged, especially where tokens are involved, by determining how much the patient will pay for the product or event. For example, if a patient will pay three tokens for a cigarette but not for a cup of tea, we can assume the cigarette is of greater reinforcing strength, and hence probably be more effective in a treatment programme. Another way of determining strength is to set a number of products or a list of events in front of the patient and let him choose which he prefers among them.

The type of behaviour to be reinforced may also be an important factor in determining which reinforcer to use. Work skills and domestic tasks appear to be most effectively reinforced with tokens for most patients, whilst with social behaviours, more natural social reinforcers seem to be the case. This may be a reflection of our culture where money is the 'reward' for work and social reinforcement the reason we behave in socially acceptable ways.

A patient must be *motivated* to acquire the reinforcer. It is unlikely a patient would behave in ways to obtain a cigarette if he already had a packet of 20 in his pocket, or strive to acquire a meal when he had just eaten his dinner.

Finally, the *size* of the reinforcer given may also determine effectiveness. We have discussed the importance of giving small 'bits' of a reinforcer when repeated successful behaviour is required to avoid satiation. However, when a behaviour will not be immediately repeated (e.g. having a bath, arising, sweeping the corridor, ironing a dress) and especially during the initial stages of a treatment programme, giving a large amount of the reinforcer contingent upon appropriate behaviour will be more effective than small amounts. Let the patient know he has done well, and he is more likely to behave that way again.

CONTROL OVER THE REINFORCER

Where reinforcers are not under the control of the therapist the possibility of effective treatment is slight. Lack of reinforcer control occurs mainly under two conditions: (1) where people involved with the patient or programme do not co-operate, and (2) where the patient can find ready access to the reinforcer.

To avoid the former, two conditions have to be met. First, all staff involved in the treatment must know the progrramme in detail and carry it out consistently. Secondly, co-operation must be obtained from the patient's relatives or visitors. One patient's husband regularly visited a patient and brought money and cigarettes, and because these were reinforcers for the patient, she would take little interest in any programme designed to help her. Though many attempts were made to persuade the husband to co-operate, his refusal effectively meant nurses had no control over the reinforcers, and treatment under these conditions cannot hope to succeed.

Patients can gain ready access to reinforcers–

(*a*) from others in their immediate environment. We may often see patients 'pestering' domestic staff, porters or other patients for cigarettes or matches. If a patient succeeds in obtaining the cigarette he is likely to adopt a similar behaviour when next he requires a cigarette as his behaviour has been reinforced. Explaining to these people the reason for the patient's programme can often help to keep the reinforcer under therapist control. Stealing may be another way of gaining access to reinforcers, and methods of reducing the possibility of this occurring have already been discussed.

(*b*) through their availability to the patient. A number of potential reinforcers may be found for a patient but cannot be used because they are freely available to the patient. For one aggressive patient, playing the piano was to be made contingent upon him being quiet during the day.

However, as the piano had no key, the reinforcer was freely available to the patient. For treatment to be effective, those involved in the carrying out of the programme must be in control of the reinforcers.

A frequently expressed criticism of using reinforcers in treatment programmes is that they are nothing more than acts of bribery. However, bribery by definition means, 'money or other goods offered to procure (often illegal or dishonest) an action in favour of the giver; or to pervert the action or judgement of another person by giving gifts or other inducements with intention to corrupt'. Bribery thus appears to involve two factors: (1) the motive or purpose of the act, and (2) the method or the way the act is performed.

Motives. When material incentives are used in behavioural treatments, they are used to promote socially acceptable and moral behaviours approved by society, and therefore the intention of the therapist cannot be regarded as an intention to corrupt or to pervert the patient's actions or judgement. Neither does the therapist gain material favour from the successful outcome of his procedures, for his income is usually dependent on the carrying out of treatment rather than the nature of its result. However, if treatment is successful, the therapist and, hopefully, the patient will both receive congratulations. The therapist from colleagues and the patient from relatives and friends.

Methods. In behavioural treatment material incentives are never given (in part or in total) *prior* to the performance of a desired behaviour. They are given only *after* the patient performs the specified behaviour under treatment—behaviours which are meant to improve his skills. Acts of bribery often involve part payment prior to the behaviour as a strong inducement to proceed with it, and do not involve teaching the receiver of the material incentive any new skills but rather the misuse of existing skills.

Chapter 12

DEVELOPING INITIATIVE

When we say a person has 'initiative', we usually mean he is not only *capable* of starting and completing a number of behaviours independently, but he actually *does* so. A frequent criticism of many long-term patients living in hospital is they 'lack initiative'. This means that though they are considered to be capable of carrying out many behaviours, they never start to perform them unless they are repeatedly reminded to do so by the nursing staff.

Lack of initiative can be regarded as belonging to the group of behaviours termed 'behavioural deficiencies'—the behaviours which patients do *not* do, and which the majority of people do perform without constant prompting from other people. Behaviours such as getting out of bed in the morning, washing, dressing and coming for meals, are some of the typical basic behaviours which patients *regularly* fail to perform unless a nurse is around to issue the appropriate instructions at the time they need to be carried out.

If a patient has the ability or skill to perform the particular behaviour associated with his initiative problem but fails to put it into operation, we may find the root of his deficiency lies more in the quality of the nurse–patient relationship and the environment in which he lives, rather than the presence of any psychiatric symptoms. By directing our attention to these two aspects of the problem, the environment and the nurse–patient relationship, we may find a solution.

Before investigating these aspects, however, we must be aware that an overall statement about a patient such as, 'He lacks initiative', is not very helpful. We need to know the specific behaviours in which initiative is absent before we can attempt to promote the initiative associated with those particular behaviours.

If a general criticism of 'lacking in initiative' was directed at us, we would regard it as unfair and unjustified. We might admit we carried out certain activities more frequently than others, and even confess there were some behaviours we rarely performed at all on our own initiative. We would certainly deny, however, that we lacked initiative. A man may lack initiative in seeking a job, yet show a great deal of initiative in going regularly to his club to play snooker and drink beer. This equally applies to patients. A mute patient who fails to wash or shave himself, does not fasten his shoelaces, or come for his medication without being told to do so, often shows a remarkable degree of initiative in obtaining a cigarette from a fellow-patient without speaking a word. It is obvious that patients are very much like other people in the matter of initiative; never completely devoid of it, but highly selective in the areas in which they practise it.

From these behavioural examples it can be readily understood that certain activities are more likely to be self-initiated if there is some incentive associated with their performance. Knowing about the value of reinforcers as motivators will provide us with a valuable aid to be used when planning treatment programmes to develop initiative.

A suggested working definition of initiative is 'the ability of a person to perform actions which result in an *attempt* to achieve a specific goal without *unsolicited aid*'. This definition emphasizes that attempting the behaviour is more important than the achievement of the goal. Though the behaviour must be self-initiated, it does not rule out the possibility of the person voluntarily seeking the aid of another; such as asking questions or seeking advice which may help him to complete the behaviour successfully.

Before any form of initiative behaviour can occur there must be:
1. a problem,
2. a search for a solution to the problem, resulting in a decision, and
3. an action as a consequence of the decision.

A problem can be regarded as a stimulus which triggers off energy directed at solving the problem. The problem can be a major or a minor one. Being irritated by an insect on the face and being trapped in a room which is on fire share common characteristics—they both require urgent decisions and immediate action.

If there is a failure to acknowledge or recognize that a problem exists, then the consequent behaviours of solution finding, decision making and action, cannot occur. Many of our patients have been in hospital a great number of years and have consequently been deprived of the opportunity of having such 'problems'. Patients have been protected from even those problems of the simplest day-to-day kind, such as choosing which clothing to wear, deciding the time to go to bed, or when to bathe. Their problem is, in a sense, *not* having problems. The remedy is to structure the environment so situations do arise which create problems for such patients.

One of the most simple yet effective situations that can create problems for some patients is produced by nurses not prompting the patient to behave in a certain way. Thus we can then measure the patient's own effort at solving his problem.

In order to simplify the assessment of patients, we can classify their initiative problems into two groups.

Group I
Those problems which are related to personal self-care activities such as hygiene, clothing, meals and all other behaviours associated with daily routine life. These behaviours involve little more than short-term planning.

Group II
Those problems which are more complex and relate to patients who no longer have any problems listed in the Group I category. The nature of their problems is concerned with longer term planning, decision making and communication with other people. The type of situations in which their initiative needs to be tested and developed, relates to seeking outside employment, finding a place to live, planning for a holiday and budgeting for future basic domestic and personal needs. Because of the diversity of these Group II behaviours and their exclusive association with particular patients, assessment charts tend to be specially designed for individual patients.

Patients with Group I initiative problems are mainly concerned with the more repetitive types of behaviour and, because these behaviours are less in number than those in Group II, lend themselves more readily to assessment charts which can be designed for the use of a great number of patients.

As in the case of all behavioural therapy programmes, the behavioural problem is measured before treatment commences. This 'baseline' measurement is used to find out how bad the problem is as well as to identify the specific areas in which initiative is lacking.

The 'Daily Initiative Rating Chart' (*Fig.* 12), consists of a checklist of daily routine events experienced by patients. Each day, for at least 10 consecutive days, nurses rate the performance of a particular patient and at the end of each day total the points scored. A high total score obviously indicates a very severe problem.

A particular routine behaviour can also be checked *across* the chart to identify specific initiative problems. The chart has deliberately not been completed in order to highlight the main problems. Item number 5 on the illustrated chart indicates a severe initiative problem. Items numbered 11, 16, 21, are less severe and may respond to treatment more easily than the previously mentioned behaviour. On the other hand, it is clear that on Item 1 the patient was out of bed on time without being prompted on 3 (30%) occasions. From this analysis it is clear the patient can perform the behaviour but on most occasions fails to do so. The implication for treatment, therefore, would be to build upon this asset.

Name: _____

Key: Performs without prompting or assistance (0)

Performs with prompting or assistance (1)

Performs with continual prompting; carried out for

patient by staff; or not carried out at all (2)

Items not applicable, or not rateable (N/A).

	Dates									
1. Out of bed	2	2	1	0	1	1	0	2	0	1
2. Washes	0									
3. Shaves	0									
4. Dresses	0									
5. Makes bed	2	2	2	2	2	2	2	2	2	2
6. Tidies room or dorm. area	0									
7. a. Sits at table	0									
8. Breakfast b. Eats food	0									
9. c. Clears utensils	0									
10. Takes medicine	0									
11. Carries out ward task	1	1	1	1	1	1	1	1	1	1
12. a. Sits at table	0									
13. Dinner b. Eats food	0									
14. c. Clears utensils	0									
15. Takes medicine	0									
16. Carries out ward task	1	1	1	1	1	1	1	1	1	1
17. a. Sits at table	0									
18. Tea b. Eats food	0									
19. c. Clears utensils	0									
20. Takes medicine	0									
21. Carries out ward task	1	1	1	1	1	1	1	1	1	1
22. Joins in recreation	0									
Total	7									

Fig. 12. Daily initiative rating chart..

Treatment should focus upon *increasing* the frequency of the behaviour he already has in his repertoire.

Two patients with apparently similar problems will very rarely, if ever, respond in a similar fashion to identical treatment programmes. Whatever the problem, whoever the patient, treatment in order to be effective must be tailored to the individual.

The first step in any treatment is to set a target level. A *target behaviour* is the behaviour we are trying to build into the patient's repertoire. The *target level* or goal, on the other hand, is the level (or standard) of behaviour we desire and hope the patient will achieve with the aid of treatment. Thus the target level for someone who talks to himself may be no observed occurrence of talking to self in 10 successive observations. For a patient who is consistently very late arriving for meals, the target level might be set at being on time for two out of three meals a day.

The exact level at which a target is set is important. It is not always necessary or desirable to achieve 100% performance or perfection. A certain amount of talking to ourselves is acceptable in the community; so is a degree of untidiness in dress, a sleep-in on days we are not working, or an amount of rubbish in our pockets. We may be sometimes in danger of setting targets too high, beyond a reasonable level for the patient. Apart from setting the final goal or target level, it may be necessary to set up sub-targets, or intermediate goals. This involves breaking down the target behaviour into steps or sequences and attempting to treat each sub-target separately, building up towards the final goal. One patient, for example, when asked a question adopted such odd behaviour patterns that his answer became almost inaudible. Analysing his behaviour carefully revealed that when he answered a question he would (1) turn away from the other person, (2) cover his mouth with his hand and (3) shuffle his feet.

These three components of his odd behaviour were taken as sub-targets so treatment was aimed first at (1). When this was successfully treated it was combined with (2) (covering his mouth with his hand), so two components of behaviour were being treated. Successful completion of these two meant the third component (3) could be added and treatment focused on all three components until the final target of answering and conversing with others appropriately was achieved.

As treatment progresses, it may become apparent that the target level initially chosen is too high or too low and needs lowering or raising respectively. There is no reason why target levels should not be changed provided a consistent measurement technique is used, and changes are kept to a minimum.

When a target level has been set, the means to achieving this is called treatment. The simplest method of treatment is to concentrate on those occurrences when the patient behaves appropriately and to reinforce these. Thus reinforcement is made contingent on desirable behaviour. Let us take, for example, the patient who was out of bed on time without being prompted on 30% of occasions. Though his behaviour is in the most part undesirable, there are occasions when he behaves appropriately. If we reinforce him on those occasions when he is out of bed on time without being prompted, he will be more likely to behave in this way again. When he does so we can say his behaviour is increasing in frequency and that we are treating his lack of initiative of not arising on time.

This is the basic premise for most treatment programmes—to reinforce the patient on those occasions he behaves appropriately. However, the majority of programmes, in addition, also concentrate on reducing the patient's undesirable behaviour. This we may do by using an extinction procedure, so on those occasions the patient performs in an inappropriate way, he would not be reinforced in any way. We call this *differential reinforcement*. The patient is not deprived of any reinforcing event, but the reinforcers are redeployed in a more systematic fashion which motivates the patient to behave appropriately.

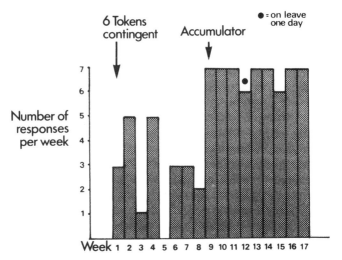

Fig. 13. Increased response in an arising programme with the introduction of an accumulator.

One interesting development in the search for techniques to increase the frequency of behaviour, is the *accumulator.* This is a system whereby a patient can earn increasingly greater amounts of the reinforcer for each consecutive successful attempt at the appropriate behaviour. One patient with a problem in arising, and who would initially rarely get up in time for breakfast, failed to markedly improve his behaviour when six tokens were made contingent upon arising before 7·10 a.m. Thus an accumulator was introduced. This involved reinforcing the patient's response on the first day with three tokens if he was up by 7·10 a.m., on the second day with six tokens, the third nine tokens and so on until on the last day of the week, if he had responded appropriately on the previous six mornings he could earn 21 tokens for being up on time. However, if he failed to arise on any day, the whole procedure would start again from the beginning, so he would be reinforced with three tokens for his next appropriate response. *Fig.* 13 indicates how this patient responded to the accumulator, reaching a 100% level in the first week it was introduced and continuing for a number of weeks at this level.

An accumulator can also be applied on a daily basis with some behaviours. Denture wearing is one behaviour with which this technique is suitable, checking the patient a number of times throughout the day and increasing the amount of reinforcer given for each consecutive appropriate response.

Where the reinforcers used in treatment programmes are tokens, there is an important question to decide upon before instigating treatment.

Should payment (or reinforcement) be all or none, or graded? The all or none method involves a patient either earning, let us say, all six tokens for being out of bed by 7·00 a.m., or none of the tokens if he fails to be out of bed by this time. Behaviours which are 'black or white' cases like this are appropriately reinforced with the all or none method. However, where the patient's behaviour can be assessed along a continuum from desirable to undesirable, graded levels for the reinforcer are more appropriate. Thus from none to six tokens may be made available to a patient for doing a domestic task, say washing the dishes. Should the patient perform this task to the best of his ability he would receive all six tokens. If on the other hand his performance was not quite so good, he would be reinforced with five tokens and so on. In this way the size of the reinforcer given is equated with the patient's performance until if the patient refused to do the task he would not earn any tokens. Graded payment has the advantage that the patient is reinforced for whatever attempt he makes which helps to establish these behaviours, and also to provide a base upon which further desirable responses can be shaped.

Our baseline measure of a patient's behaviour may indicate that he is unable to perform the behaviour at all without prompting (e.g. item 5 on the Daily Initiative Rating Chart, *Fig.* 12). Such an example of an initiative problem concerned a patient who consistently failed to come to the trolley for his three-times-a-day medication. The nurse decided to give the patient two tokens each time he came for his tablets without being prompted. In addition to the tokens he would, of course, be complimented each time he achieved his target. The nurse–therapist's problem was, how to get the patient to start coming for his tablets in the first place in order to give him these rewards.

This treatment programme continued for many weeks with very unsatisfactory results. Prompting of the patient by a nurse seemed to be the only way the patient could obtain his medication. But prompting also meant he would never receive any material or social rewards.

The nurse responsible for this patient's treatment decided to see what happened during the period when the medicine round was conducted. After each patient had finished his meal and helped to clear the table of used crockery and cutlery, he approached the nurse dispensing the drugs and received his prescribed medicine. One of the few exceptions to this pattern of behaviour was that of our special problem patient. Like all the other patients, he carried his used crockery to the food trolley, but after depositing his utensils on the trolley, he always walked over to the lounge area, sat down in a particular armchair and leisurely lit his cigarette. Meanwhile, the nurse giving medicines waited the 5 minutes extra time allowed the patient to remind himself to come for his tablets. The nurse waited in vain, and once again had to call him for his tablets.

There is little point in continuing a treatment programme which consistently shows poor results. Neither is it fruitful to blame the patient for treatment failures. Poor results are more likely to be due to faults in the design of the treatment rather than faults in the patient. As a consequence of the nurse's observations and analysis of the patient's behaviour, she decided to embark on a fresh approach to the problem. At the next mealtime (breakfast on the following day), and before the medicine round took place, she stationed herself in the path of the route regularly taken by the patient on previous occasions. Standing directly in front of the patient's favourite chair, she waited for him to finish his breakfast. Sure enough, as the patient got up from his chair with his cup, saucer, plates and cutlery, he first walked towards the food trolley and then headed directly for his armchair. The patient suddenly discovered he had a problem. Blocking the path to his chair was a nurse. As he side-stepped to make a detour around this human obstacle, the nurse side-stepped in unison. With a puzzled look on his face at this nurse's peculiar behaviour, the patient said, 'What's up?' 'Haven't you forgotten something, Fred?' A brief pause followed by 'No, I've not forgotten anything'. 'How about your tablets then?' replied the nurse. After a quick 'Oh!' Fred turned away and went directly to the nurse giving the tablets. He did not, however, receive any tokens or praise for his action.

At lunch-time the nurse–therapist was already in position when Fred took his familiar route. As soon as Fred saw the nurse, he turned around and went directly to the nurse giving out the medicines and, for the first time, received his tokens as well as receiving complimentary remarks from the nurse doing the medicine round for coming to get his tablets without being told to do so by the nursing staff.

In effect, Fred had been prompted to get his tablets when he saw the nurse standing in front of his chair. He obviously remembered his experience with this nurse after breakfast and had associated the nurse's presence with 'getting his tablets'. The quality of the prompting had, however, changed and become more refined. In place of a direct vocal instruction (a verbal prompt), it had now become a visual stimulus (a non-verbal prompt), which had triggered his behaviour to go for his tablets.

The nurse–therapist attended every meal period for five consecutive days. At each meal time she gradually moved away from Fred's armchair, increasing the distance away from Fred as he came each time to the food trolley to deposit his used crockery. The nurse not only increased her distance but gradually changed directions until, by the end of the week, the nurse was no longer in the dining area, and therefore not visible to Fred.

Despite the nurse's absence, Fred continued to come for his tablets without any prompting at all—verbal or non-verbal. The nurse had used the procedure known as 'fading'. That is, having established herself as a stimulus, which had helped to remind Fred to get his tablets, the nurse had now successfully faded her presence from the scene enabling Fred to continue his habit of coming for his medicine without the aid of any further 'prompting' stimuli. The material and especially the social reward could now, and hopefully, later maintain his behaviour.

In developing a patient's initiative we are not attempting to teach him a new behaviour, but rather to extend and improve the skills of his existing behaviour. We try to do this by providing him with the most appropriate settings and conditions which will enable him to have frequent opportunities to practise these skills.

The influence of environmental conditions is particularly important in assisting or hindering initiative behaviours. Sometimes the rearrangement of these conditions alone may be sufficient to allow particular forms of initiative to be expressed and, eventually, established. In other cases, some form of stress situation may be the most suitable way of developing initiative.

Chapter 13

DEVELOPING 'NEW' BEHAVIOURS

Training is a process of learning. In order to be able to read, swim, cook or play cricket we undergo training. The various skills we have acquired as a nurse are learnt through training. Almost every behaviour we possess has been learnt at some time, and how well we perform the behaviour depends upon how well we have been trained.

Training involves changing behaviour patterns. Either a new behaviour is added to the person's repertoire or an existing one is modified. Either way, change comes about through learning. In this chapter we will discuss some of the training techniques which have proved useful in maximizing learning in the chronic patient.

Some patients fail to possess a behaviour in their repertoire. For example, they may lack speech of any kind (mutism), or fail to carry out a ward task such as setting a table. In such cases using differential reinforcement (i.e. reinforcing desirable behaviour and not reinforcing undesirable behaviour) is not appropriate for there is no desirable behaviour to reinforce. What we need are techniques which will help to develop new behaviours in the patient's repertoire.

TECHNIQUES USED IN DEVELOPING BEHAVIOUR

What can the patient do? As when we explore means of developing a patient's initiative, we first have to find out what the patient is capable of doing, for he may never have been given the chance to show his skill of a particular behaviour since his admission to hospital. This we may do either by: (1) *Withdrawing* staff help from the situation—for instance by leaving a patient to attempt dressing himself, or by not responding to a mute patient's gesture for a cigarette, to see if he will say anything, or (2) *asking* the patient to perform the task. We might ask him to set the table, or write a letter to his relatives, for example.

Whatever the patient's attempt, or lack of attempt at performing this behaviour, it gives us an indication of his level of performance.

Approaching the problem this way has certain advantages over jumping headlong into teaching the patient a behaviour. These are:
(*a*) It saves time, i.e. the patient is not taught things he may be capable of doing already.
(*b*) Any attempt by the patient provides a base on which to build the behaviour.
The main techniques used in building up behaviours are:
1. Instruction
2. Imitation
3. Shaping

1. Instruction

In our everyday life we frequently learn new behaviours by following instructions. For example, we learn how to fill in tax forms, take medication, or use the self-service petrol pump and launderette by reading instructions. Once we have performed the behaviour on a couple of occasions, we no longer need to refer to the instructions—we have learned a new behaviour.

Instructions can be either of a verbal or written nature. Verbal instructions, if the behaviour is carried out straight away, permit the instructor to give immediate feedback and provide extra information or alternative ways to tackle a problem if at any point the patient fails to grasp the idea. Written instructions, in comparison, allow patients to go at their own pace, and can be carried from one place to another, so reducing the need to memorize instructions.

Instructions should be given in ways which make them easily comprehensible. This often means making written instructions simple, easy to follow and, where possible, aided with diagrams. Verbal instructions are easier to understand where they are given in 'bits', rather than whole masses of detailed information. The translating of an instruction into action is a process requiring the patient's attention. Thus where instructions are lengthy or detailed the capacity of a patient to keep these in memory and act on them may easily be exceeded, especially if we consider he may also have problems in concentration. We all know how easy it is to forget simple verbal instructions such as the direction to some place we have never been to before. The general rule therefore is not to 'overload' the patient with information, but to make instructions as simple and clear as possible.

Instructions can be very quick and effective in teaching certain behaviours to high-level patients. Where a patient already possesses some of the basic skills necessary to carry out a new behaviour, all that may be required to teach him the behaviour is to give certain basic instructions which will help him coordinate the skills. For example, a patient who is familiar with kitchen utensils, is able to wash up and knows where the stores are kept can be taught to clean out and stock up a kitchen cupboard by following instructions such as, 'Remove all objects from the cupboard, throw away empty boxes and jars, wash down the shelves, ensure there are three jars of pickles, three of jam, etc'. On the next occasion the patient comes to clean out and stock up this cupboard he may need little if any instruction in how to do it.

Instructions become very laborious and inappropriate when teaching behaviour from the beginning, or in teaching complex behaviours such as speech or the methods involved in physical exercises. Some behaviours such as fastening a button may appear quite simple but are very difficult to teach using instructions alone, for they require fine manual dexterity. Instructions may be of use in starting off 'simple' behaviours. Ayllon and Azrin, for example, had a number of patients on their ward who failed to pick up eating utensils before a meal. After simply instructing the patients in how and when to pick up their implements (before collecting the meal), 40% of them started to perform the behaviour regularly. When reinforcement was introduced in addition, all the patients began picking up their utensils.

2. Modelling (Imitation)

We have the capacity to incorporate long chains or sequences of responses into our behavioural repertoire simply by observing someone else making these responses. Imitative or observational learning plays a part in the acquisition of many behaviours including social skills, swimming, dancing and many, many others. Nurses learn various ward procedures through imitation, first observing qualified nurses perform the behaviour and then attempting to carry out the behaviour in a similar fashion. It may be that patients on long-stay wards learn some of their institutionalized behaviour by observing what other patients do.

As a treatment technique, imitation involves the nurse (or model) showing the patient a particular sequence of behaviour and then reinforcing him if he successfully copies the behaviour. It is a particularly useful and effective technique with schizophrenic patients, because their difficulty in handling 'abstract' information can be avoided by the 'concrete' behaviour demonstrated by the model.

Learning through imitation involves three stages:

(a) *The modelling of the behaviour* by the nurse while ensuring the patient is looking at the demonstration. She may direct the patient's attention to a particularly difficult aspect of the behaviour by supplying comments like, 'Watch this', or, more specifically, 'See how I hold the brush with two hands'. Sometimes the behaviour may have to be broken down into its elements or components and these demonstrated in turn, building up the complex behaviour by advancing onto further components when the patient has mastered the previous one. For example, for a very withdrawn patient, the behaviour of mopping may require breaking down into three components: holding the mop, the act of mopping and the squeezing of the mop in a bucket. If the patient finds three components too complex, then each component may have to be broken down again into even simpler components.

(b) The patient is given a chance to *imitate* the nurse. He begins by trying a response which appears similar to that made by the nurse. His first attempts may be rather crude as this is a very complex process for the learner, involving the translating of a visual perception (what he sees performed) into a motor response (his attempt at copying).

(c) *Feedback.* After his first attempts at copying a demonstrated behaviour, the patient needs to perfect his response by trial and error. This is achieved by reinforcing those responses which increasingly approximate those of the model, and by feedback. If the action has clearly identifiable consequences, as in mopping up a pool of water or dressing oneself, then the patient can obtain feedback from the environment. Whether the behaviour has such observable results or not, verbal feedback is necessary, both in order to inform the patient where he has excelled, and to direct his attention to those aspects which still require modifying.

Modelling requires a great deal of co-operation from the patient, for the best results obviously occur where the nurse is imitated immediately and the actions are 'fresh' in the patient's memory. For some patients this co-operation cannot be achieved until they have been taught how to imitate. The starting point is then to establish what in fact a patient can imitate. For example, though a patient may not be able to speak, the starting point in the treatment of this problem may be to reinforce simple motor acts—something he is capable of copying. The imitation of words may then be established by reinforcing an increasing range of acts which gradually include verbal elements. Speech has been introduced into patients' repertoires in this way by systematically modelling and reinforcing the patient's attempts at standing up, touching his mouth, opening his mouth, wagging his tongue, blowing out a match, coughing, and saying 'cat'. After the establishment of one or two imitated words (e.g. car, catch, chair) the basis is laid for further speech development.

Modelling can be used to help develop a wide range of behaviours. Eisler and Hersen have demonstrated the use of modelling in teaching social skills deficits to institutionalized patients. Training consists of:

(i) The nurse presenting an interpersonal situation. For example she may set up a situation with:

'You are standing in a queue waiting for your medicine when someone comes up and gets ahead of you in the queue.'

Another nurse, acting as the queue jumper says, 'You don't mind if I go ahead of you?'.

(ii) The patient responds to the situation.

(iii) The nurse provides *feedback* about the adequacy of the patient's response. It is always advisable first to praise those aspects of the patient's performance which were appropriate or an improvement on a previous performance. This is then followed by drawing the patient's attention to how he might improve on his response.

(iv) The nurse may model the appropriate response.

(v) The patient has a further attempt.

Modelling of social skills is important for the long-stay patient as it appears social competence is one of the best predictors of adjustment to life outside hospital for chronic psychiatric patients.

This procedure has been applied in both individual and group contexts. It can be a highly effective and rapid method of developing appropriate behavioural responses. Modelling is at its most effective when:

(i) The patient is reinforced for performing the demonstrated behaviour. Long-stay patients can acquire new behaviours through observation without necessarily being reinforced, but the combination of modelling and reinforcement of imitative responses is much more effective than the presentation of a model only.

(ii) The nurse who models is 'liked'. People tend to imitate better the people they like which again reflects the importance of nurse–patient relationships.

(iii) The patient already has components of the modelled behaviour in his repertoire. Behaviour is more readily imitated when an individual already possesses elements or rudiments which can be tied together to form the more complex behaviour which is being modelled.

On a ward concerned more with therapy than with custodial care, there are ample opportunities for imitative learning. Those patients functioning well in such an environment act as a model to others, who see how the formers' progress is met with all forms of reinforcement from the staff.

3. Shaping

A behaviour which does not occur in the patient's behavioural repertoire can be gradually shaped out of his existing behaviour by reinforcing responses which proceed in the desired direction and not reinforcing other behaviours. The word *shaping* is borrowed from sculpture where a block of clay is gradually shaped to the desired results. Because the process of shaping involves successively reinforcing behaviour which increasingly approximates to the desired behaviour, it is sometimes called *successive approximation*. Both terms are equally appropriate, but shaping has an active connotation emphasizing the therapist's involvement in reinforcing first one and then another response, whereas

The reason we might use shaping to establish a behaviour is again illustrated with mutism. A chronic patient who has been mute for years is not likely to start spontaneously uttering words so that we can reinforce him. First we need to teach him to utter a word and this can be achieved through shaping, by reinforcing him for the slightest approximation towards speech, such as movement of the lips and grunts.

The steps in shaping involve:

(a) Ensuring the behaviour can in fact be carried out. If because of brain damage or some other physical deficiency there is no possibility that a given response can be emitted, then any attempt to shaping is a waste of time.

(b) Define the initial and end behaviour (targets). A vague definition makes it difficult for the nurse to know what she is aiming to achieve. The target behaviour may be broken down into steps or sub-targets. For example, the target may be to teach a patient to work for 30 minutes during occupational therapy. Should the patient show no signs at all of working, the first sub-target or step might be set at teaching him to hold the tools (e.g. hammer and nail, or sandpaper), and then successive steps towards the target may be using the tools, working for a minute, for 5 minutes and so on, gradually increasing the length of time working at the task.

(c) Reinforce the existing response. It is important for the patient to see that a reward is available, so reinforcement should follow the occurrence of an existing response which has a component related to the target behaviour. Such an existing response in a mute patient might be eye contact, or in the patient at O.T. it might be showing curiosity in the tools set before him. We may try to establish an initial response in the absence of any appropriate behaviour by providing an example of a behaviour which he may imitate (e.g. the mute patient may be given a sound to imitate).

(d) Reinforce variations in the direction of the target behaviour. For example, patients with almost inaudible speech may be reinforced at those times they speak a little bit louder. The mute patient may be reinforced for his approximation of the model's cough.

(e) Raise requirements gradually. The behaviour should be established at each sub-target before requirements are raised. A mute patient should make consistent audible coughs before we move on to the next step of requiring a word. If we move too rapidly from one step to another the behaviour already shaped may extinguish. Alternatively, if we continue to reinforce at one level for too long the behaviour may become so firmly established that it becomes difficult to move the patient along to the next step. The size of the step required of the patient is also important, for if it is too great, the patient may never achieve the level and therefore never receive reinforcement. If this occurs, the size of steps needs to be reduced so less is required of the patient in order to gain reinforcement. The size of each step which can be taken obviously depends upon the individual concerned, but too small a step does not usually cause problems because the chances of an appropriate response and hence of reinforcement increase.

An example of shaping may serve to illustrate these steps. A patient who had been mute for a number of years was first reinforced with a piece of chewing gum for eye movement towards the gum. Once this response was established the nurse held up the gum and waited for a movement of the patient's lips before giving it. This step was followed by one requiring a sound like a croak and then the patient was asked to say 'gum', and was reinforced for approximations to this sound. When the patient uttered the word 'gum' he went on to make further verbal responses.

As can be seen in this example prompting or modelling ('Say gum'), increases the chance of the patient performing an appropriate response. Shaping is a time-consuming technique but can be useful where other methods such as instruction or modelling fail to have the required effect; and as such it is more appropriate with the lower level of patient where certain behaviour is non-existent.

ADDITIONAL PROCEDURES

Teaching behaviour to a patient does not just involve the carrying out of one of the techniques outlined above. All these methods should involve additional procedures which when used correctly facilitate training and help the patient learn new behaviours. These procedures are:
1. Prompting
2. Praise and informational feedback
3. Practice
4. Fading

Prompting

Prompting is something we all do to certain degrees. For example, a husband may prompt his wife to pay the gas bill, or she may remind him not to forget the tickets for a dance. Prompting is a form of giving assistance or cueing a person into what is expected of him.

Prompting can be particularly useful in the early stages of training. It is economic in the sense that the patient is helped to perform a behaviour reasonably quickly without the nurse having to wait for it to occur.

The various forms of prompting are:
1. Physical prompts—helping the patient perform correctly by giving him physical assistance. For example, we might show a patient the correct way to hold a sweeping brush by placing both his hands in the appropriate place.
2. Gestural prompts—this is where we indicate to the patient what might be expected of him, by means of gestures. Both physical and

gestural prompts are often accompanied by verbal prompts, so the behaviour comes to be associated with a verbal label.

3. Verbal prompts—these were discussed earlier (p. 66) where it was suggested that they can either be directed, when the action desired of the patient is expressed (e.g. 'Isn't it time for occupational therapy?'); or undirected, where the patient is given a prompt that something is expected of him but he is not told what (e.g. 'Perhaps there's a better way of doing that'). He is left to discover what it is he should be doing, and thus has to start thinking about his behaviour.

Though prompting is useful in initiating behaviour, it should be reduced in a systematic way when the behaviour is established. The methods of doing this were discussed in Chapters 6 and 12.

Praise and informational feedback

We should never forget the importance of praising appropriate behaviour whenever it occurs, or of providing informational feedback whether the behaviour is appropriate or not. Along with verbal feedback, information may be provided through visual cues (e.g. looking at one's appearance in a mirror after dressing); or by taste (e.g. sampling the food one has cooked).

Practice

Practice is useful in two respects:

1. It aids better and smoother performance. A skilled man works at a task smoothly, and has plenty of 'time' because he is able to anticipate events. In contrast, a person learning a skill cannot work smoothly because he occasionally does things wrongly, and doesn't have the same 'time' to carry out the behaviour because he is unable to anticipate what is likely to occur next. During practice, therefore, we should concentrate on specific parts of a behaviour the patient performs badly, and on repetition of the behaviour so he may start to anticipate events.

2. Practice also reduces the chance of forgetting. It might appear that events with a verbal nature (e.g. a joke, a new address or telephone number) are more easily forgotten than motor behaviour (e.g. riding a bicycle, swimming), but this is not, in fact, the case. There is no real difference in the retention of either verbal or motor behaviour, the apparent difference being in the amount we practice each. Verbal items which are practised can be remembered well, as for example a favourite quotation or the words of a favourite song.

Fading

This is the process whereby prompting is gradually removed until the patient is able to perform the behaviour under his own initiative. This was discussed in Chapter 12 with relation to developing a patient's initiative.

Fading can be applied both to the use of verbal cues so that the patient learns to carry out the behaviour spontaneously under his own initiative, and to the nurse's presence so that the behaviour is performed in her absence.

Establishing the greeting response in a patient's repertoire illustrates the first of these fading techniques—that of fading a verbal prompt.

Nurse	*Patient*
1. Approaches patient and says 'Hello'	
2. Approaches patient and says a faint 'Hello'	If patient says 'Hello' he is reinforced.
3. Approaches patient and just mouths the word 'Hello'	
4. Approaches patient and remains silent	

The fading of a nurse's presence can be demonstrated with a female patient who would not leave the ward unaccompanied by staff. The patient was eventually taught to use buses and go into town for the first time in a number of years. This was achieved through supporting the patient in new situations and then fading the staff's presence. Each stage was practised a number of times:

1. Patient and nurse left the ward for a social in the hospital grounds.
2. Patient and nurse went to town on the bus, the nurse paying the fares. They looked round the shops and returned by bus, the nurse again paying the fares.
3. Patient and nurse went to town, the nurse watching as the patient paid her own fare on the bus.
4. Patient went alone by bus and met the nurse in town.
5. Patient went alone, did some shopping and came back alone.

Fading is a useful technique for developing the patient's spontaneity, when his response is tied to some stimulus, such as a verbal cue from the nurse or a particular person. However, it may be an overlaborious method with the higher level patient and for such the instruction, 'Now you try it without my help' may be sufficient.

Chapter 14

PUNISHMENT

There are a number of techniques which can be used to reduce undesirable behaviour, some of which have been discussed already, such as extinction (p. 62), and some of which are discussed in Chapter 15. However, the technique most people associate with reducing behaviour is *punishment*. After all, it is the most frequently encountered method of 'stopping' behaviour in modern life. We are punished at home and at school as a child if we do anything wrong, reprimanded at work if we begin to 'slack', fined if we commit a driving offence, and so on.

Whilst punishment has many ethically loaded connotations, it can be defined as a behaviour procedure very simply. Punishment occurs when a behaviour is weakened by an event which follows it in time. However unpleasant it may seem, a stimulus is not defined as a punisher by its intrinsic qualities, but rather by the effect the stimulus has on the preceding behaviour. Only if a particular stimulus weakens or terminates behaviour which it systematically follows is the process called punishment. Spanking a child therefore is only a punishment if it produces a reduction in the behaviour on which it is contingent. Spanking which does not produce a change in behaviour is not a punishment, and may well reflect the frustration of the parent rather than a real wish to control or change behaviour.

Some people so strongly oppose the use of punishment that they prefer not to explore the topic at all. Our position is more moderate, in that we will attempt to describe the procedures but also provide considerable cautionary information. It is our belief, that since punishment procedures lend themselves to overuse and abuse, they are best employed as a last, rather than a first attempt to remedy a problem.

There are two types of punishment which differ quite markedly in technique. These are punishment by aversive stimulation and by withdrawal of positive reinforcers.

AVERSIVE STIMULATION

This is a procedure whereby a painful or unpleasant event is presented contingent upon the occurrence of an undesirable behaviour. An example of such aversive stimulation might be smacking a child for his misdemeanours. With long-stay patients the most common occurrence of such punishment is verbal reprimands from staff when a patient's behaviour falls short of what is expected. In one study a patient with auditory hallucinations was given a shock box and was instructed to carry it around and shock himself immediately the voices began and until they ceased. The occurrences of hearing voices dropped to zero. Another patient's 'nipping' behaviour was treated by slapping his hand every time he tried to nip a member of staff.

The effect of this type of punishment is far from conclusive. There is evidence to suggest that under appropriate conditions punishment can operate to reduce the frequency of behaviours quickly and effectively. However, in treatment settings these appropriate conditions can hardly ever be established because the number of factors needed to ensure punishment is maximally effective is immense:

1. There must be no possible escape for the patient.
2. Ideally, punishment should be awarded to every incorrect response, which means almost continuous observation. If punishment is given intermittently, there is the chance that undesirable behaviour will be reinforced on occasions and thus become more resistant to change.
3. As with positive reinforcement, punishment must be given immediately the undesirable response occurs.
4. Punishment should be quite intense. If the punishment is not intense enough at the outset, the patient will learn to adapt to gradual increases in intensity.
5. Extended periods of punishment should be avoided.
6. An alternative response should be made available where the patient can be reinforced.
7. The patient should be informed of the reasons for not engaging in the punished behaviour.

Unless the patient is willing to be involved in a punishment programme, as the patient who shocked himself whenever he experienced hallucinations, then these conditions can never be met in a ward programme and hence the effectiveness of punishment techniques will be minimal.

Professor Skinner has suggested that although punishment may initially suppress behaviour, this is only a temporary suppression, as once the punishing agent is withdrawn behaviour reverts to its previous level. This we know from our personal experience—when the school-teacher goes from the room, children no longer continue writing but begin talking and playing. When a patient is reprimanded for eating his meals with his fingers he may pick up his knife and fork, but come the next meal he will most probably begin eating his food with his fingers again. When conditions cannot be controlled, then punishment only temporarily suppresses behaviour. When the punishing agent is not present, or the punishment procedure removed, undesirable behaviour has a tendency to reappear.

Why then is punishment used so much? Well, as a practical mode of behavioural control, punishment produces results fast, much faster than by extinction. A telling off or a smack will stop a child's undesirable behaviour immediately. However, the behaviour will emerge at a later time, because punishment does *not* eliminate it from the person's behavioural repertoire, but merely suppresses it.

Where punishment may be used to some effect depends upon what happens during the brief period following the punishment. During the time the person's undesirable behaviour is suppressed, positive aspects of his behaviour need to be reinforced and strengthened. However this should never be accepted as a motive in the use of punishment. Alternative methods which aim to modify the patient's behaviour rather than suppress it, should be sought. Some of the reasons why punishment by aversive stimulation has little effect in establishing new behaviour include:

1. Punishment generates emotional behaviour both in the punisher and the recipient, and these unpleasant feelings are not conducive to learning.
2. The person being punished for his maladaptive behaviour is not taught any other alternative and appropriate way to behave. He is left to discover more appropriate ways on his own, and so without guidance he either behaves the same way again in similar conditions or tries out new ways of behaving which may also be inappropriate.
3. Punishment does not remove the positive stimulus maintaining the behaviour. If it is nurse's attention or specific situations which maintain a patient's behaviour, then the presence of these conditions will spark off the behaviour when the punishing agent is not present. The advantage of extinction lies in the fact that it removes the stimulus maintaining the behaviour and thus weakens the response.
4. Punishment procedures are difficult to implement because there is usually a time delay between the patient doing something wrong and being discovered, if at all he is discovered.

Side-effects

Not only are punishment techniques less effective in changing behaviour but they may have various side-effects.

1. Punishment generates unpleasant or aversive conditions, and so the patient learns to *avoid* or *escape* from the situation or nurse presenting the punishment. For example, a patient may run away

or learn to avoid contact with nurses, making the administration of punishment even more difficult. It also leads to a deterioration in nurse–patient relationships because patients learn to 'fear' a particular punitive nurse or nurses in general. This produces tense and maybe hostile atmospheres which are certainly not conducive to learning. In the interests of overall learning it is better to keep the environment positive in tone rather than negative.

2. The person applying the punishment is reinforced for using punishment, for when she applies it, the behaviour is temporarily suppressed so she sees that she can stop behaviour through using this method. She therefore comes to use punishment more and more often as it appears an effective way of altering behaviour. However, because it is only temporarily suppressed, the behaviour will reappear and she thus has to punish the behaviour more and more, often intensifying the punishment in the process.

3. Punishment may produce counter-aggression. The patient slapped for persistent 'touching' of others may hit back at the punisher, causing an intensifying of the punishment by the punisher. A spiralling interaction may develop in which both emit increasingly severe punishing behaviour.

WITHDRAWAL OF POSITIVE REINFORCERS

By this technique something appealing to the patient is taken away because he engages in undesirable behaviour. Positive reinforcers are withdrawn, contingent upon the occurrence of inappropriate behaviour. This may be accomplished in two ways: (1) response cost procedures and (2) time out.

Response cost involves the removal of a positive reinforcer from the patient. It costs the patient to behave in an inappropriate way. It may involve the forfeit of material reinforcers (such as cigarettes), the deprivation of privileges (such as refusing usual use of a single room), or fining tokens contingent upon undesirable behaviour. Many of these are traditional but primitive ways of controlling behaviour. For example, we often see a patient 'paying' for leaving the ward without permission, by being put in pyjamas and dressing-gown for a day or two.

Many of the criticisms levelled at the use of aversive stimulation as a form of effective behaviour control can be applied to response cost methods. They can easily become overused and produce a 'fine mad' situation where the patient is made to pay for every minor infringement through the loss of reinforcers. Punishment should be limited in its use to those behaviours where all other efforts at modification have failed.

The implementation of response cost methods should involve decisions on the precise cost to be attached to each instance of the undesirable behaviour. Costs should never be decided on the spur of the moment, as anger or disappointment over the patient's behaviour will probably cause us to overcharge.

Time out involves removing the patient from a situation he finds reinforcing, when he persists with his inappropriate behaviour. The non-availability of positive reinforcers to the patient is equivalent to extinction. However, time out differs from extinction in that no positive reinforcer is available for any behaviour as long as the time out procedure is in effect. With extinction we need to know the reinforcer that is maintaining behaviour for it is this which we withhold from the patient contingent upon his undesirable behaviour. However, we can use time out without knowing the maintaining reinforcer. Because isolation withdraws so many potential sources of reinforcement it is likely that it produces a time out from access to positive reinforcement. Schaefer and Martin have illustrated the use of this technique in the treatment of persistent disruptive behaviour such as screaming, fighting, cursing, throwing objects and breaking articles. Patients who behave in this manner are often reinforced because they secure nurse's attention and thus the disruptive behaviour is maintained.

Extinction procedures such as ignoring the aggressive behaviour may not work because the patient's behaviour interferes and disrupts the general ward programme. In such cases the time out technique is useful. It involves:

(a) Escorting the patient to a quiet room so he is removed from the ward and any reinforcing situations.

(b) Making as little fuss as possible and issuing no comment to the patient when removing him. If we start to argue or discuss the reasons for placing him in time out he obtains exactly that attention which reinforces his undesirable behaviour.

(c) Ending time out when the patient is quiet or shows signs of desirable behaviour. If we allow him to return when he is still exercising undesirable behaviour we are reinforcing his behaviour.

(d) Ensuring there is a time limit so the patient is not left in a time out situation for too lengthy a period of time. There are no firm guidelines for the duration of time out, but brevity is desirable since it both minimizes the time during which the patient is removed from the learning situation and since time out is aversive, any desirable behaviour the individual engages in while in time out is paired with the aversive stimuli. Thus, in effect he would be punished while behaving desirably. Time out should not exceed half an hour, but in the majority of cases it will be much less, and may last for no more than a few minutes in many cases.

Once a patient has experienced time out a verbal comment may be enough to stop the behaviour. For example, we may say to a patient who starts disruptive behaviour at the meal table, 'Stop, or it'll be time out.'

Obviously if he continues with his inappropriate behaviour we have to act on what we say and put him in time out.

Time out is only appropriate for behaviours which are disruptive in nature—aggressiveness, shouting, throwing and so on—those which can be eliminated by isolation from other people. It is inappropriate to use time out as a punishment for not performing a specific behaviour (for example, not washing or not being prompt for medication) and for behaviours which are inherently reinforcing where the patient can reinforce himself whilst in time out (for example, self stimulation).

As time out refers to any method that removes the patient from the reinforcing environment, it may not necessarily involve him being removed to a quiet room. Standing in a corner facing the wall may be one effective method, with the proviso that should he attempt to return to the situation before a predetermined time has elapsed, he is given an additional minute in time out. Another method may involve refusing to let a patient use the ward shop, if he has been stealing. The important thing to remember is the situation from which the individual is removed must function as a positive reinforcer otherwise the technique will not be effective in reducing behaviour.

COMPARISONS (or differences!)

The difference between some of the techniques we have discussed sometimes appears to be rather hazy. In order to try and clarify these, the differences are set out in *Fig.* 14. Perhaps the most difficult to distinguish between are withdrawal of positive reinforcement from extinction and between aversive stimulation and negative reinforcement.

Withdrawal of positive reinforcement differs from extinction by the fact that in the former a positive reinforcer, *not* necessarily the one maintaining behaviour, is *removed.* In contrast, during extinction a reinforcer that *is* maintaining the behaviour is *withheld.* Let us consider a patient who expresses delusional ideas, a behaviour which is being maintained by nurses' attention. To reduce this behaviour by extinction would involve *withholding* nurses' attention (the reinforcer maintaining behaviour) when the patient expressed delusions. However, to reduce it through the withdrawal of positive reinforcement would involve removing a reinforcer, not necessarily the one maintaining behaviour (perhaps a cigarette, or a token), from the patient whenever he spoke in a bizarre fashion.

Aversive stimulation and negative reinforcement are distinguished by the effect they have on behaviour. With the former, the unpleasant stimulus *decreases* the behaviour upon which it is contingent, whilst negative reinforcement *increases* the target behaviour because it enables the individual to escape or avoid the unpleasant stimulus. Therefore the

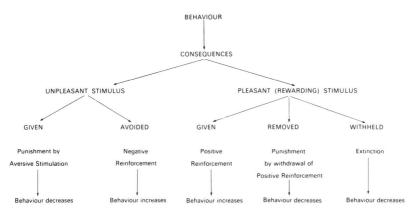

Fig. 14. All behaviour has consequences. Here the consequences (unpleasant or rewarding stimuli), the different methods of application and the effects they have on behaviour, are illustrated.

same unpleasant stimulus can be used to suppress undesirable behaviour through punishment and also negatively reinforce (increase) behaviour which succeeds in escaping or avoiding it.

In summarizing, punishment techniques are not as effective as some might suppose. As there are procedures which are equally effective in eliminating undesirable behaviour which do not involve aversive stimulation or withdrawal of positive reinforcement, as we will see in Chapter 15, it is good ethical practice to restrict the use of punishment techniques to circumstances where no effective alternative methods are available.

Chapter 15

FURTHER PROCEDURES FOR
DECREASING BEHAVIOUR

Inappropriate behaviour, as we have seen, can be reduced by *extinction*—a slow but effective method in situations where we can identify the maintaining reinforcer; or by *punishment* (averse stimulation, or withdrawal of positive reinforcers)—methods whose effectiveness in reducing behaviour is far from clear unless a number of optimal conditions are met. Other methods which can be utilized to decrease behaviour, often quite quickly, include:
1. Looking at the antecedents and consequences of a behaviour.
2. Using reinforcers in programmes designed to reduce behaviour.
3. Overcorrection.

LOOKING AT ANTECEDENTS AND CONSEQUENCES

If we are able to identify those events or stimuli which are maintaining a behaviour, and we are in a position where the stimuli can be modified, then the behaviour is also likely to change. Some undesirable behaviour is produced by situations in the environment. A patient pestering for a light for his cigarette may have no other means of obtaining one. If we supply him with matches or a lighter and teach him how to use these items, we may reduce the incidence of 'pestering'. Changing the circumstances or *antecedents* of a behaviour is instrumental in changing the behaviour on many occasions, as we reduce or eliminate the events which trigger the undesirable behaviour. Unsociable behaviour such as eating greedily may be reduced if patients are given sufficient time to eat their meals; and hoarding of 'irrelevant' objects may decrease if the patient is allowed to keep personal possessions in a safe place such as a locker with a key.

The traditional scavenging for cigarette-ends was reduced on one ward by substituting traditional coarse toilet paper, which made adequate cigarette paper, for soft toilet paper. Those patients who sought out cigarette-ends to use the tobacco in making up cigarettes with toilet paper, could no longer do this, for the soft tissue type did not make very good cigarettes. The behaviour of another patient who used to eat out of the pig bucket was modified by simply giving him more to eat during a meal. He had taken to eating from the pig bucket because he was still hungry!

By studying the *consequences* of a behaviour, we may discover why a behaviour is being maintained. Let us take a patient who is doubly incontinent. If whilst taking a baseline to see how frequently his behaviour occurs we also study what actually happens when he 'dirties' himself, we may come to an understanding of why he behaves as he does. Imagine we check him once every hour. When he is 'clean' he would obtain a tick on his chart, but what happens when he is 'dirty'? He would get a cross on his chart, but also most probably be bathed immediately and given a clean set of clothes. If we analyse what has happened we see that when he is 'dirty' the consequences are nurses' attention, a warm bath and clean clothes, but when he is 'clean' there are no such desirable consequences. He therefore receives 'reward' or reinforcement contingent upon his undesirable behaviour and not his desirable behaviour, so maintaining the former. Studying the consequences of a behaviour often reveals why the behaviour is being maintained.

The implications for treatment are obvious. Reinforcement needs to be reversed so it is contingent upon appropriate behaviour. In the above example the patient may therefore be reinforced during a toilet training programme, and given attention on the ward when he is 'clean'. However, when he is 'dirty' he should not be reinforced with pleasant consequences. He should be cleaned up, but in water which is not pleasantly warm, and given a clean set of clothes but in a neutral manner which does not convey acceptance of his behaviour.

A procedure which can be applied to some behaviour is of letting the patient experience the consequences of his behaviour. Often a patient will behave in a disruptive manner but be shielded from the consequences. Thus a patient who deliberately throws his meals on the floor is often helped to calm down and then given another meal. This reinforces his disruptive behaviour. To treat such behaviour we teach him what the consequences of his behaviour are. Thus he would be required to clean up what he has thrown on the floor. Similarly if a patient throws and breaks some of his own property, then this is lost to him, unless he makes efforts to mend it. Any appropriate behaviour such as mending the possession should be reinforced.

Patients can be taught the futility of engaging in many undesirable behaviours by showing them it is not 'profitable'. Undesirable behaviour such as stealing money, raiding the ward shop, burning dresses with cigarette-ends, and catching taxis from town and charging the fare to the hospital, have been reduced by giving the patient a 'bill'. This bill outlines what the behaviour cost and the patient is required to pay this off by earning an appropriate number of tokens before he is again allowed to use the ward shop. In a way this is a 'fine' but it is directly related to the cost of the behaviour. Thus stealing of one pound's worth of goods from the ward shop would mean the patient paying a pound back, probably by instalments with the tokens he earned for more appropriate behaviour. Thus he gains nothing from having stolen, so the consequences of behaving in such ways is no longer reinforcing and hence the behaviour of stealing will extinguish.

USING REINFORCERS TO DECREASE BEHAVIOUR

Designs for decreasing behaviour by using reinforcers include:
1. Reinforcing incompatible behaviour
2. Reinforcing reductions in behaviour
3. Reducing reinforcer dependent upon the degree of undesirable behaviour
4. Paying for the privilege of undesirable behaviour
5. Satiation

Reinforce incompatible behaviour. This means specifically reinforcing behaviour which cannot be produced at the same time as inappropriate behaviour. Two behaviours are incompatible when they cannot be produced at the same time. For example, a parent who reinforces a child for talking appropriately may find bouts of screaming decreasing because screaming is incompatible with talking.

In the treatment of patients' problem behaviours, this technique can take on two forms: reinforcement of *non-occurrence* of the undesirable behaviour, and reinforcement of *specific incompatible behaviours.*

The first of these—reinforcing *non-occurrence* of undesirable behaviour—is not concerned with teaching a particular form of behaviour, but rather it emphasizes the patient be rewarded if he does not display inappropriate behaviour. So, for example, a patient who persists in talking to himself may be reinforced for not indulging in this behaviour. This technique usually involves a time limit which may be as short as a minute to begin with, so that if a patient does not talk to himself throughout this time, he would receive reinforcement. Time limits would then be gradually extended maybe to 5 minutes, 10 minutes and so forth. Other behaviours treated in this way may be reinforcement for not lying on a bed, or not pacing the corridor. The initial time limit has to be one the patient can reasonably achieve and this is then gradually extended. Such an approach emphasizes the elimination of a behaviour from the patient's repertoire but is not concerned with what takes its place, as long as it is not the particular undesirable behaviour in question. Thus, a patient reinforced for not talking to himself may achieve the required response and gain his reward by being mute during the specified time—also not a particularly appropriate behaviour.

Reinforcing a *specific incompatible behaviour,* on the other hand, is concerned with what takes the place of the undesirable behaviour. If we are dealing with a behaviour problem such as talking to self we might require the patient to speak to other people (appropriate behaviour) in order to gain reinforcement. Such an approach does not involve time limits but concentrates on reinforcing behaviour which is both appropriate and incompatible. It is therefore concerned with both building up appropriate behaviours and decreasing undesirable behaviours rather than concentrating primarily upon the latter, as arises with just reinforcing the non-occurrence of a behaviour.

Reinforcing incompatible behaviour lends itself to the treatment of a number of behavioural handicaps. Destructive patients may be reinforced for constructive acts such as might occur during a group activity session, loud and verbally aggressive patients may be reinforced during moments of quiet or appropriate speech, and patients who incessantly pace the corridor may be reinforced for periods of sitting reading, knitting or doing a crossword.

Reinforce a reduction in behaviour. It is possible in some situations to reduce the magnitude of a behavioural problem by reinforcing attempts the patient makes to reduce the behaviour. Obesity is a frequently encountered problem amongst long-stay patients, and one potential solution is to put the patient on a diet. However, where the incentives of food and 'doing nothing' (inactivity) override that of being slim, then the patient will not be motivated to lose weight and may consequently sabotage the diet by obtaining extra food either 'legally' (spending their money on sweets and cakes) or 'illegally' (stealing food or eating out of the waste bucket).

However, a patient may be motivated to lose weight if he sees himself as involved in the treatment programme. In the treatment of obesity the incentive may be, for example, a large number of tokens for every one pound of weight lost, at a weekly 'weighing in' session. Such an approach puts the onus on the patient and it is he alone who is responsible for losing weight, not some diet imposed upon him by other people.

A further example of this approach involves a patient who wore an excessive amount of clothing. Treatment involved her having to lose weight by discarding some of the clothing before being allowed into the dining room—food being a reinforcer for her. On successive occasions she was required to weigh less and less, until the stage was reached where she began wearing an acceptable amount of clothing.

Another patient hoarded on average six old newspapers in his jacket pockets during the baseline. On some occasions, therefore, he would have more than six old papers in his pockets, but on others he would have less. Treatment of this problem involved reinforcing him on those occasions where he had six or less newspapers in his pocket. We reinforce initially at the 'average' so the patient becomes aware reinforcement is available. Gradually the criteria is made more stringent so he is reinforced only on those occasions he has five or less papers in his pockets. By gradually extending the criteria in this way, at those times when he is easily capable of achieving the criteria, we are reinforcing reductions in his behaviour.

Reduce reinforcer depending upon the degree of undesirable behaviour. As this design usually involves delay of the reinforcer, it is only suitable for the higher level patients who are fully aware of the programme's details. Reinforcement is set at a level, and is available in full to the patient if his behaviour is appropriate throughout the day. However, should he behave inappropriately at any time, the size of the reinforcer is reduced by a predetermined amount, and whatever is left is then given at the end of the day.

For example, a patient may be told that 30 tokens are his if he does not swear at staff or patients throughout the day. Each time he is heard swearing, he loses two of the tokens, so that in effect it costs him to swear. At the end of the day, the cost of his swearing is deducted from the 30 tokens, and he is given the remainder.

Paying for the privilege of performing undesirable behaviours. Here the patient is given a choice as to whether he wants to behave inappropriately or behave normally, always assuming the patient is capable of knowing the difference. If he elects to behave inappropriately it costs him. This differs from a fine, for payment occurs before the behaviour is performed, whereas with a fine, payment is a consequence of doing something inappropriately—it comes after the behaviour.

Ayllon and Azrin used this approach with a patient who persistently ate his meals messily. He did this to gain nurses' attention, and he could eat normally when he desired. The treatment was to charge three times as much if a meal was to be eaten messily. Before each meal a nurse asked the patient whether he wanted to eat the meal appropriately, which would cost the usual amount, or whether he would like to eat it messily which would cost three times as much. If he chose the former and then proceeded to eat it in a messy fashion, the meal was removed. In this way the patient's behaviour improved to the point where he regularly ate his meals in a more appropriate fashion.

Satiation. We have talked about increasing behaviour by following it with a positive reinforcer, but if an activity or behaviour is followed by, or associated with, too much of the positive reinforcer, then the behaviour will decrease in frequency. This phenomenon is probably familiar to all of us, especially at Christmas time. Turkey, from being well appreciated with the Christmas dinner, begins to lose some of its attraction after the turkey salads, turkey sandwiches and turkey broth that arise on the following days. We become satiated with turkey.

Though not a technique which can be applied widely, satiation has been used to reduce certain behaviours such as delusions and hoarding. With the former a patient attended sessions each day where she had to talk for 30 minutes about her delusional beliefs. After a period of time the patient tried to avoid going to the session and it was reported the amount of delusional speech fell slightly on the ward.

However, the classic example of successful employment of a satiation technique comes from Ayllon's work. One of his patients persistently hoarded between 19 and 29 towels at any one time in her room. Nurses would regularly clear these out, only for there to be a similar number in her room on the next check. Ayllon queried that nurses in removing the towels were paying attention to the behaviour and hence may have been maintaining it. He therefore instructed nurses to refrain from removing any more towels from the room. The patient was given more towels on a non-contingent basis until after 3 weeks she had accumulated 625 towels in her room. At this point the patient announced she had had enough and began removing the towels herself. Thereafter she began to keep only one or two towels in her room, a behaviour which was maintained for over a year.

Satiation is the overuse of a positive reinforcer, which causes the reinforcer to lose its 'strength' until it becomes neutral or even aversive to the patient. Thus the patient's behaviour stops being reinforced. As we have seen, behaviour which is followed by no reinforcement is an extinction procedure, and behaviour followed by aversive stimulation is a punishment procedure, both of which work by decreasing behaviour. However, because satiation is often a time-consuming and not very practical technique, its use is very much restricted.

3. OVERCORRECTION

Overcorrection was first described by Foxx and Azrin, being a procedure applied contingently to behaviour which requires decreasing or extinguishing altogether. They described two basic components:

1. restitution
2. positive practice

An example of *restitution* for someone who threw his food on the floor would be to require him to clean and wash the floor and then to clean other parts of the dining room. This goes one step further than the procedure of letting the patient experience the consequence of his behaviour (page 155). With restitution he is not only required to restore the situation to how it was before he threw his meal on the floor but, in addition, to make the environment superior to how it was originally, before the inappropriate act.

Positive practice involves the practising of new, more appropriate alternative responses, generally with between 10 and 30 repetitions of the same response contingent on each episode of the inappropriate behaviour. For example Azrin and Wesolowski used positive practice to treat a patient who sprawled on the floor. He was required each time he was found lying on the floor to practise several times getting up from the floor and sitting in a chair. This method is considered more socially acceptable than many aversive procedures because the consequences of the inappropriate behaviour used with overcorrection follow 'logically'.

The two components of overcorrection can be applied in combination (restitution being applied first followed by positive practice) or as distinct and separate treatments.

Foxx and Azrin have insisted that certain aspects of training must be present before treatment can be classified as overcorrection:

1. requesting the patient to refrain from the inappropriate behaviour

2. physically preventing him from further emitting the behaviour

3. minimizing positive reinforcement and requesting his involvement in restitution or positive practice with a neutral tone and as little emotional expression as possible

4. performing graduated guidance, which consists of physical prompting to encourage the patient to perform the required response.

5. relating the treatment directly to the inappropriate behaviour (e.g. cleaning the dining area for throwing food)

6. introducing overcorrection immediately following the inappropriate behaviour

Overcorrection is being used as an alternative to many traditional aversive procedures. Early uses of overcorrection involved treatment of a wide range of maladaptive behaviours such as self stimulation, floor sprawling and, in children, nocturnal enuresis.

With long-stay patients, aggressive behaviour has been treated using overcorrection. Matson described a patient who threw objects, such as bits of paper, into the faces of other patients and staff. He treated this through overcorrection by first discussing the incident with the patient and having her formulate an apology including regrets and a promise not to repeat the behaviour (verbal restitution). The patient was then required, for 5 minutes, to pick up litter from the floor and put it into a waste bin, so teaching an appropriate way to handle litter. Graduated guidance was attempted only if the patient refused to carry out the overcorrection.

Chapter 16

REVIEWING PROGRAMMES

After treatment has begun it is essential to continue monitoring the patient's behaviour and obtain up-to-date records of his progress. At regular and frequent intervals all those concerned and involved in the patient's treatment programme should meet to discuss his progress. Where there is little evidence to suggest the patient is performing any better than he was during the baseline, or where there are signs of deterioration in his behaviour, it is clear the treatment is not working. It would be inappropriate to carry on with the programme unaltered in such circumstances for it is unlikely the patient will suddenly begin to respond. Rather, it would be more appropriate in such a situation to find out why the treatment programme is ineffective. Occasionally it turns out the programme is not ill-designed or inappropriate, but that other extraneous factors are limiting its effectiveness. Therefore before radically altering a treatment programme, we might ask two questions:

1. 'Is the patient capable of responding?' We need to consider whether the patient is physically capable of behaving in the required way. Though this should be investigated before setting up the treatment programme sometimes factors not immediately apparent may be found to be inhibiting the patient's progress. For example, one patient's attempts to get up on a morning at the appropriate time were hindered by excessive night sedation. When medication was gradually reduced the patient began achieving a much better perfomance on the programmme.

2. 'Are staff carrying out the treatment correctly?' We have discussed the problems of inconsistency in carrying out a programme and the disastrous effects it may have on a patient's behaviour. All the members involved in the treatment must be aware of the definition of behaviour and the methods of carrying out treatment. Often at reviews such inconsistencies become apparent. A graph may plot the general trend of a patient's behaviour, but a chart may help to identify where the problem

lies. Where ratings taken by one nurse consistently differ from measurements taken by all the other nurses it may indicate the nurse is unclear as to what or how the measuring should be done. On a female appearance checklist the item 'hoarding under clothes' was generally understood to refer to whether a patient accumulated rubbish on her person underneath her clothes. One nurse, however, thought it was an item to determine whether the patient hoarded *under-garments* in her handbag or locker. Both are problems with long-stay patients, but this patient was being rated for different problem behaviours depending upon which nurse was rating. The inconsistency became apparent by looking at the appearance chart, because the patient did in fact hoard underneath her clothes, and therefore obtained a tick on most ratings except when the ill-informed nurse rated the patient.

If the answers to these two questions are positive the treatment programme may require modification. Alterations might include:

1. *Relaxing the criteria level.* A patient on a programme to increase his speed of working may be reinforced when he completes his work in 30 minutes. However, if this criteria level is too strict the patient may never achieve it and hence never be reinforced. By extending the criteria level to, say, 40 minutes there will be more chance of him being reinforced. Later when he regularly starts to finish his work in 40 minutes, the criteria level can be made more stringent by reducing the time limit to, say 35 minutes and then finally to 30 minutes.

2. *Increasing the size of the reinforcer or adding other reinforcers in combination.* Where tokens by themselves are not sufficient to increase a patient's arising behaviour, giving a cup of coffee in addition to the tokens can markedly increase the patient's response. Alternatively some patients may be helped by a *bonus* scheme where an extra privilege is made contingent upon the patient's responses reaching a certain level. For example, one incontinent patient, reinforced hourly (12 times a day) when dry, could earn an additional sum of tokens at the end of the day if he achieved 8 out of 12 dry hourly sessions. With improvement, the criteria was raised gradually until eventually to earn his bonus tokens, he was required to stay dry at all 12-hourly checks.

3. *Involving the patient more.* This may include providing more visual feedback on a patient's performance in the form of charts or graphs freely available for all to see; self-recording through patients keeping their own chart up to date by means of ticks and crosses or stick-on stars; or by negotiating the terms of treatment with the patient. With higher level patients the terms may be discussed and agreed, so a 'contract' is signed by both patient and staff which states that the patient will receive certain specified reinforcers, if he behaves in particular ways.

4. *Changing the reinforcer.* Only one out of 12 patients regularly attended group activity sessions on time when tokens were the reinforcers, but when the mid-morning cup of coffee was made

contingent upon being prompt at the session, the other 11 patients began attending on time more regularly.

5. *Focusing tokens.* This involves changing the pattern of distribution, from a small number of tokens given for many behavioural problems to a large number of tokens for a particular behavioural problem. That is, concentrating tokens on the problem causing most concern. For example the pattern of reinforcement may be changed:

	Rising on time	2 tokens	
	Appearance	2 tokens	
From:	Dry bed	2 tokens	To: Dry bed 10 tokens
	Bed made	2 tokens	
	Taking medication	2 tokens	

Because of individual differences and the specific differences of each behavioural problem it is difficult to predict the response of a patient to a particular programme. Reviewing progress then becomes all-important, since modifications small or large are a necessary part of the treatment if success is to be achieved and stagnation avoided. The alterations do not stop when behaviour has improved and the target level reached. Then comes perhaps the most difficult part of the programme. The success of a treatment programme is not measured solely by whether the patient improves his behaviour to an acceptable level but by whether once this has been achieved the following take place: (1) the desirable changes in behaviour accomplished in one situation are extended to other situations—*generalization* and (2) the contingencies can be removed so that eventually the behaviour may be maintained and performed spontaneously in the natural environment. The gradual reduction and eventual complete removal of the reinforcer is called *weaning*, or 'thinning out'.

GENERALIZATION

What may happen when a behaviour has been learned is that it becomes tied to the situation in which it was acquired. This applies especially to one-to-one situations where a nurse spends time with a patient away from the ward setting teaching a specific behaviour. There is then the potential problem that although the patient may acquire a behaviour, he performs it only in the room where treatment occurred, and only when the particular nurse is present. The behaviour is 'tied' to stimuli such as the room and the nurse, because the patient has never been reinforced for the behaviour in other situations or by other people. Transfer of this learning to other people and other appropriate places needs therefore to be taught. This is called *stimulus generalization.*

Generalization, whereby behaviour learned in one setting appears in another appropriate setting, is a natural phenomena. If this were not so we would have to continually learn, for example, how to open a door every time we came to one we were not familiar with. Behaviour is more likely to generalize to a novel setting if it is similar to the setting in which the behaviour was learned. People find it relatively easy to drive a 'new' car because behaviours we learn in driving our own car are useful in helping us adapt—the behaviour generalizes. However, if we tried to drive a bus, though some generalization would occur, it would take longer to master the driving because it is less similar to our own car.

Where patients behaviour is tied to one person or one situation, transfer of learning has to be taught. The patient who has been taught how to speak in a one-to-one session needs to learn to speak in other situations and to other people. This is done through reinforcement of appropriate behaviour, perhaps in a group meeting or generally on the ward. Treatment programmes involving all staff and carried out on the ward avoid this generalization training. However, the successful ward programme still has to ensure the behaviour is transferred from the treatment situation to the real life situation. Procedures which increase the chances of generalization and which hence avoid continuous relearning in the real life situation are listed below.

Using natural reinforcements

Social reinforcers should be used in treatment wherever possible for they are more 'natural' and are apparent in the real life situation. One exception is behaviour concerned with work. As the 'natural' reinforcer for work is usually money in our society, then tokens may be of particular use with behavioural problems concerned with work. When material reinforcers or tokens are used, then as soon as possible they should be substituted for either 'real currency' or gradually faded and substituted for social reinforcement. This process is not easy. It can lead to excessive social reinforcement in an attempt to compensate for the loss of material reinforcement, which is both unnatural and may lead to dependence on social reinforcement. The problem is eased in some situations where improvement of a behaviour opens the door to many 'natural' reinforcers. Speech is one example, for after the patient develops it to a reasonable level he is in a position to ask for things and converse though probably at an elementary level. This leads to him being naturally reinforced, when others respond to him verbally.

One obese patient who rarely washed and had untidy clothes improved with token incentives. She was taught to use make-up and began to attend socials and dances with other patients. She began to enjoy these events immensely and found a male friend which provided sufficient incentive for her to remain clean and tidy even when tokens for good appearance were removed. Her behaviour had come under the influence of more 'natural' reinforcers.

Simulate environmental conditions on the ward

The closer the treatment situation resembles the natural environment, the greater are the chances of generalization. Thus only those behaviours which will be of use to the patient should be taught him. It may be appropriate to teach a patient to use the hot water geyser in the hospital, but on discharge will this skill be appropriate? More likely he will need to know how to use a kettle.

The ward may be able to adapt its routine and procedures to simulate events in the community and hence make ward life and 'outside life' more comparable. Meals routinely served up without involving the patient in any choice may alternatively be served cafeteria style. The patient may then learn to pick up a tray, tell the server what he wants and even possibly pay for the meal once selected (if on a token economy ward). This has been done on one ward and patients have then been able to 'use' self-service cafeterias in the community appropriately. Role playing may be carried out so that the patient experiences a job interview, a supermarket situation or a 'pay as you enter' bus before he attempts the real thing. On token economy wards, patients learn to budget their money and enter saving schemes. Even the token can simulate 'real currency', plastic decimal coinage being a method of familiarizing patients and enabling them to go into the community and spend money appropriately. These are just a few examples of the way a ward can simulate the world outside hospital, to help the behaviours learned on the ward generalize to outside life.

Teach patients in the natural environment

Exposing patients to the natural environment is the real test of treatment success. Patients may have been taught how to use money, eat appropriately or open a bank account on the ward, but only when the patient experiences the real situation can we tell if the behaviour has generalized. Nursing support is necessary in the initial stages of generalization when reinforcement should be given for appropriate attempts but with the nurse gradually fading from the situation.

WEANING

Newly acquired behaviour cannot be forever tied to programme contingencies but needs to come under the control of the patient himself. However, frequently the level of behaviour is only maintained while contingent reinforcement is in operation. Thus once reinforcement is withdrawn, behaviour tends to fall to its previous baseline level. Though this may demonstrate the effectiveness of reinforcement, it does not demonstrate that problem behaviour can be treated, for therapy should show changes which are maintained beyond the treatment conditions

themselves. If a change in behaviour only occurs during treatment, whereas removal of the conditions results in a loss of treatment effects, therapy cannot really be said to have taken place. Sudden withdrawal of reinforcers produces extinction. The patient finds himself not being reinforced for previously reinforced behaviour and hence the behaviour will extinguish, and most possibly return to the baseline level. However, behaviour can be maintained at a high level by a gradual planned procedure. In this way newly acquired behaviour can become permanent rather than being susceptible to the reinforcement conditions prevailing at the time. Methods of weaning include:
1. Reducing the reinforcer
2. Linking or chaining behaviours
3. Delayed reinforcement
4. Schedules of reinforcer

Reducing the reinforcer
This involves a gradual reduction in the amount of reinforcer given to the patient. As many workers have stressed, this should be in combination with an increase in emphasis on more natural reinforcers (social and privileges) so that eventually the latter will suffice to maintain the behaviour. This technique is particularly useful where natural reinforcers are incentives to the patient. With high-level patients they often are, and consequently the approval of nurses and others, or the chance to go into town when they look neat and tidy, become a sufficient reinforcer to maintain behaviour. However, the more withdrawn patient may not find natural 'reinforcers' as reinforcing, especially since by definition such patients tend to avoid social contact. Once the strength of a reinforcer is reduced, as when the reinforcer is reduced in size, it may not be potent enough to maintain the behaviour. Other reinforcers for the patient such as doing nothing, being stronger and also incompatible with desirable behaviour, reduce the chance of appropriate behaviour. Hence this method of weaning may not be appropriate for some patients. However, where it is appropriate the simplicity of the method makes it very attractive to use. The programme is only minimally altered, since the patient is still reinforced immediately after every response he makes, but the size of the reinforcer given is reduced.

For example, one patient would rarely bathe himself and required a prompt from the nurse to have a bath. During the baseline when prompts were removed, he bathed only once in 2 weeks. Treatment consisted of reinforcing him with eight tokens on completion of a bath, but his behaviour failed to improve. Making 20 tokens contingent upon having a bath increased his behaviour until he began bathing on average 5 days a week. Once his behaviour stabilized at this level, weaning consisted of gradually reducing the tokens, so he would receive 18 tokens for a bath.

After a while, 16 tokens were made contingent upon having a bath, at each stage being careful not to reduce the tokens by too large a step. Gradually the size of the reinforcement was reduced until none at all was given, without any deterioration in his behaviour. In a token economy programme, where a number of patients are reinforced with tokens for a number of behaviours, the success of gradually reducing the number of tokens for a particular behaviour may lie in not reducing the patient's total income. Therefore when tokens for a particular behaviour need to be reduced, the tokens should be loaded on to another behaviour problem the patient is being treated for. This links up with the previously presented idea of 'focusing' or concentrating tokens on one problem rather than spreading them thinly over a number of problems.

Linking (or chaining)

This involves the building up of behaviour by reinforcing the completion of a number of consecutive responses. Basically there are two varieties:

(*a*) Where the same behavioural responses are linked so that consecutive occurrences of appropriate behaviour, not interspersed by inappropriate behaviour, are required before reinforcement follows.

Linking similar behaviours, e.g. two consecutive responses

	1	2	3	4	5	6	7	8	9	10
Patient's response	✓	O	✓	✓	✓	O	✓	✓	✓	✓
Response reinforced				★				★		★

KEY: ✓ Appropriate response   O Inappropriate response

An example may help to illustrate this technique. Consider a patient who is reinforced with three tokens each time he gets up on time in the morning. When he reaches a 100% level (arising each morning of the week) and remains at this level for a few weeks, the weaning stage may require him to get up for two consecutive days before he receives his reinforcement.

The successful accomplishment of two consecutive responses will then lead to three and so on until if he continues to maintain this high level of response, the patient may be required to get up on time all 7 days to earn the reinforcer. If he fails on one day, then the counting would start again, his next appropriate response being counted as the first.

The procedure can also apply to behaviour repeated a number of times per day. For example, should a patient receive reinforcement for working a session of 30 minutes at O.T., and he reaches a target of working most sessions, then two 30-minute sessions may be linked, then three and so on until all sessions have to be completed before reinforcement is available.

(b) Where different behavioural responses are linked so sequences of behaviour may be built up. Two behaviour problems which have been separately treated may for example be wearing dentures and keeping the wardrobe clean. When the patient is able to perform both adequately they may be linked so that he is required to do both to obtain reinforcement.

Linking two different behaviours

		1	2	3	4	5	6	7	8	9	10
Patient's responses	Behaviour A	╱	╱	╱	╱	o	o	╱	o	╱	╱
	Behaviour B	╱	o	╱	╱	╱	o	o	╱	╱	o
Response reinforced		★		★	★				★		

It may be preferable but not essential to link behaviours which occur in sequence, such as those involved in early morning routine. For example, when each behaviour can be performed adequately the stages in linking the separate behaviours may be:

Stage 1 (treatment)
        (a)   Rising before 7.00 a.m.   4 tokens
        (b)   Dressing correctly   4 tokens
        (c)   Washing face and neck   2 tokens

Stage 2 (linking 2 behaviours)
        (a)   Rising before 7.00 a.m.
  and (b)   Dressing correctly   } 8 tokens

Stage 3 (linking 3 behaviours)
        (a)   Rising before 7.00 a.m.
        (b)   Dressing correctly   } 10 tokens
  and (c)   Washing face and neck

Separately treated behaviours can thus be 'chained' together to form a sequence of behaviour. The size of the reinforcement given at any stage in linking separate behaviours is again largely at the discretion of the therapist but should eventually be reduced gradually when the sequence of behaviours can be performed adequately.

Because with linking procedures, whether any response is reinforced depends upon the patient's immediately preceding behaviour, the nurse has to keep adequate records. Nevertheless it is a particularly useful way of extending behaviour often providing an incentive for the patient to work towards, for he knows exactly what he must achieve if reinforcement is to be his.

Delayed reinforcement

This involves accumulating the reinforcers (usually tokens) earned for various behaviours and presenting them in a lump sum at a later time. Such techniques reduce the patient's dependency upon reinforcement through being taught not to expect immediate payment after each appropriate behaviour. Delayed reinforcement is especially useful with domestic ward tasks and work performance, probably because being akin to 'wage' payment it reflects the association between work and payment which is central to our culture.

The patient will normally be socially reinforced and told how much he has earned for each occurrence of appropriate behaviour. The earnings are then totalled up and presented as a 'wage' or lump sum. Again the method may not be appropriate for the very withdrawn patient for he may fail to respond to the social reinforcement and the delay restricts his awareness of what specific behaviours the 'lump' reinforcement is for. From the nurse's point of view delayed reinforcement increases the work load, for as well as reinforcing each individual behaviour socially, she has to keep a record of how much the patient has earned.

The length of delay can obviously vary but, in a systematic plan, the delay would be gradually lengthened. Ward tasks which are originally reinforced immediately may be reinforced with tokens at the end of the day, then perhaps on every alternate day, gradually extending the delay until a patient works for a week before receiving his wage.

Again the point at which to change the programme is critical, for if the delay is increased too early or in too large a step, the patient's behaviour will deteriorate. Constant monitoring helps to avoid this and lengthening the delay should only be attempted when the patient's earnings become stabilized at a relatively high level.

Schedules of reinforcement

During treatment, desirable behaviour is usually reinforced on a continuous basis, where every appropriate response is reinforced, whilst inappropriate responses are extinguished. However, on a schedule of reinforcement only a certain proportion of the appropriate responses is reinforced. The responses selected for reinforcement are done in a predetermined way so that the patient is unaware which of his responses are likely to be reinforced, but knows that at least some will be. The nurses follow a 'schedule' or programme which gives details of the responses to reinforce. There are three types of schedule: (*a*) random; (*b*) fixed ratio; and (*c*) variable ratio.

Random schedules. A predetermined set of responses to be reinforced is chosen at random so the patient does not know whether he will or will not receive reinforcement at any check.

Random reinforcement

	1	2	3	4	5	6	7	8	9	10
Patient's response	✓	✓	○	✓	○	✓	✓	✓	○	✓
Predetermined plan	●			●	●		●			●
Response reinforced	★			★			★			★

Fig. 15 shows a random reinforcement programme for various items of appearance with five patients. All five patients were capable of performing well on these items and the programme was introduced in an attempt to maintain their behaviour. Each patient was required to remain tidy throughout the day, for the check could be made in the morning, or the afternoon, or not at all (number 0), and could be made on one of three pairs of items (number 1, 2 or 3). Thus a patient would be reinforced with four tokens if he performed well on the two items which were checked at that time; two tokens if he did well on one and not on the other item; or no tokens if he performed badly on both items. There is thus an incentive for the patient to maintain his appearance. From a nursing point of view such a schedule means that the nurse does not have to refer to any previous behaviour in order to reinforce at any particular time, but simply has to stick to the predetermined plan or schedule.

Fixed ratio schedules. Here reinforcement follows the occurrence of a number of responses. For example, a fixed ratio 3 (F.R. 3) schedule means the patient is reinforced after he makes three appropriate responses.

Fixed ratio schedule

	1	2	3	4	5	6	7	8	9	10
Patient's response	✓	✓	○	✓	✓	✓	✓	○	✓	✓
Response reinforced (F.R.3)				★			★			

Numbers	Items	Tokens
0	No spot check	Nil
1	Hair tidy	2
	Shoes polished	2
2	Shirt clean	2
	Tie clean and neat	2
3	Jacket clean	2
	Trousers clean	2

Plan for week commencing ....

Patients	M am	T pm	W pm	T pm	F pm	S am	S am
J. Brown	2	1	3	1	2	0	0
A.Tomms	2	0	2	1	1	3	2
F.Webb	2	1	1	0	2	3	1
J.Smith	1	3	2	0	3	2	2
L.Wood	0	2	2	3	0	1	3

Fig. 15. Random appearance item check..

He can make undesirable responses, but only appropriate responses count. Here the nurse working to the schedule has to keep a check on the patient's previous behaviour—she has to count back to ensure she is reinforcing the right occurrence. The schedule can gradually be extended so that an increased number of responses is required by changing the schedule to say a F.R. 4—every fourth response, then F.R. 5 and so on. Very few schedules can in practice be perfectly adhered to because much behaviour both appropriate and inappropriate goes undetected by the staff, and because patients may understand the schedule and 'fiddle' the system.

Variable ratio schedules. These schedules work in a similar way to fixed ratio, but instead of every response being reinforced, reinforcement follows a variable set of occurrences of the behaviour.

Variable ratio schedule

	1	2	3	4	5	6	7	8	9	10
Patient's response	✓	✓	✓	✓	o	✓	✓	✓	✓	✓
Response reinforced		★					★			★

(V.R.3 - 2nd, 4th, 3rd)

For example a variable ratio 5 schedule (V.R. 5) means that on average the behaviour is reinforced on the fifth occasion. It may be the fourth response, then the sixth and so on, but on average it will be every fifth response. The ratio too can be extended gradually so the patient is performing more and more without reinforcement.

Though schedules are often difficult to apply, they can be very effective methods during weaning, for behaviours reinforced under schedules of reinforcement do not extinguish as easily as those reinforced under a continuous schedule, when reinforcements are withdrawn. This phenomenon is again probably familiar, for every time we put a coin into a coffee machine, we are being continuously reinforced with a cup of coffee. However, if the coffee did not appear we might bang and kick the machine or call the operator, but we would be unlikely to put more than one more coin in—our behaviour has been extinguished (rapidly!). Now consider the fruit machine which pays out or reinforces only infrequently (on a variable ratio schedule). We merrily put coins in the machine, unaware of when the pay-out may be, but our behaviour does not extinguish, as long as we are occasionally rewarded (or run out of money!)

Quite a number of patient's behaviours such as cigarette-end hunting are reinforced on a variable schedule. Because they will occasionally find a butt-end this reinforces their searching and hence the reason why it is very difficult to break the behaviour. Behaviour learned under variable ratio schedules are very difficult to extinguish.

FOLLOWING UP PROGRAMMES

Once a new behaviour has been established and the reinforcement phased off, a check on the behaviour should be kept for a few weeks to defect any deterioration. Even later at 3 months, 6 months and 1 year after the end of weaning, checks may be made to observe for any deterioration in the long term—these are called follow-ups. In practice a follow-up is essentially the same as a baseline except that it occurs after treatment, and so needs to be conducted in a similar fashion without prompting the patient. Follow-ups are necessary if we are to know if all our efforts at treatment, generalization and weaning have been successful in maintaining a behaviour in the natural environment.

Chapter 17

GROUP ACTIVITY PROGRAMMES

There seems to be common agreement between staff working in psychiatric hospitals that all organized activities of a social or creative character are beneficial in some way to psychiatric patients. In what particular way these activities are beneficial, and in what manner they function to produce favourable results, are questions which are difficult to answer precisely without reviewing various aspects of these activities, examining the reasons given for organizing them, and assessing their relevance to patients' problems.

An activity can be used as a *therapy* or a *recreation*.

As therapy

One reason given for engaging patients in organized social activities is 'it is therapeutic'. According to our understanding of the definition of therapy, it means 'treatment'. Treatment includes identifying specific problems of particular patients, assessing the severity of these problems, prescribing programmes designed to alleviate or eradicate the problems, monitoring results of treatments in the most objective way possible and, finally, keeping records of the result of treatment.

If these conditions are fulfilled, then the selective use of an activity to assist in the treatment may be justifiably called therapeutic.

As recreation

Not all activities are therapeutic, nor is there need for all activities to be used as treatments. The majority of activities in psychiatric hospitals are not, and do not need to be, structured in this way. When the aim is simply to provide a programme of social events which resident patients can attend voluntarily, then these activities do not require further justification. Film shows, bingo sessions, dances etc. are intended to counteract boredom and to help maintain or improve the quality of life in hospital. The patients who regularly attend these functions choose to go voluntarily, have ability to take part, socially interact with other people, and generally behave appropriately. Their regular participation is sufficient evidence that the activity itself is, in some way, rewarding for them. There is no need to describe their presence at a dance as 'dance therapy', listening to music as 'music therapy', a visit to the cinema as 'film therapy', nor winning the jackpot with a 'full-house' as 'bingo therapy'. For these people it is a recreational activity—a pleasurable experience which occupies their time. The term 'recreational therapy' is therefore inappropriate.

THE PROBLEM

There are many patients who do not voluntarily make use of any of the available recreational facilities provided by the hospital. They are often described as 'lazy', 'apathetic', 'depressed', or 'institutionalized'. Whatever label is attached to them, all staff recognize these patients as having a problem. Because excessively long periods of inactivity are generally regarded as unhealthy, nurses also have a problem; the problem of what to do about these patients.

The conventional approach to the problem is to 'round up' a number of patients, call them a group, and escort them to the activity currently available. Having arrived at the location of the activity, the next problem is to get patients to participate in it. At this stage of the procedure problems become more complex. We learn in the practical situation that patients do not always immediately make use of the facilities provided. They often have to be taught how to use them. The manner in which each patient responds to this situation may vary considerably, and this adds to the problem of attempting to teach them all how to participate appropriately in the activity. It is relatively easier to get a number of patients to walk to the scene where the activity is to take place than it is to involve them in it. The reason for this is clear. When everyone responds in the same way to a single simple instruction, we can cope with a large number of people. When responses to a general instruction differ, we have to approach each person separately to find out what the difficulty is for each one before the whole group can respond in a suitable manner.

Without some form of systematic approach to this difficult situation the problems become overwhelming. One thing is certain, these patients are not taking part in any recreational activity, nor can they be seen to be involved in any well-defined therapeutic venture.

A POSSIBLE SOLUTION

The use of behavioural treatment procedures offers a systematic method of approach to many problems associated with long-stay patients. Group activity programmes add another dimension to its value as a treatment by providing appropriate settings in which these treatments can take place.

As we have seen, it is customary for those conducting behavioural treatment to analyse a particular problem and define the terms they use before rushing in to perform treatment. Before discussing the practical use of various activities in detail, it may be helpful to define the meaning of Group Activity Programmes.

A Group is a collection, a bunch, a clump or an assembly. In this particular instance the assembly is a group of people. The opposite word to 'group' is 'individual'. We can, therefore, define a group as 'a number of individual people assembled for the purpose of engaging in a specific activity, or activities'.

Activity means behaviour involving action which is purposive, is related to an ongoing event, and in which all members of the group participate. There is an ideal number of people for each kind of activity.

Programmes are a pre-planned series of events which are communicated to all members of the group in advance of the date and time they are due to take place. It is advisable that some printed record of these programmes is avilable to all participants to which they can refer before the events occur.

Group activity programmes consist, therefore, of a number of pre-planned events designed to involve patients and nurses in a variety of structured group situations. These shared common experiences provide an ideal environment in which skills related to a social interaction, communication and organization of joint projects can be practised. They attempt to cater for the physical, intellectual and social needs and interests of the patients who form the group and *are part of a treatment programme*. Though the events are planned by the people on the ward, they need not be ward-based. They can take place in any appropriate setting within or outside the hospital. Group activities are distinct from and supplementary to the ward daily routine activities which deal with problems related to the performance of domestic chores, meals, hygiene, clothing, etc. They are also distinguished from leisure periods in which patients participate voluntarily in any social activity of their own choosing.

The combination of a structured setting, a programme for teaching a variety of skills, and the social interaction between nurse and patient, is the basis of this aspect of behavioural treatment.

PLANNING ACTIVITY PROGRAMMES

When first organizing a weekly programme of group activities there may be a tendency to favour the idea of asking patients what they would like to do. This initial approach to patients who have never before experienced a regular sequence of activities for any length of time is unlikely to produce many enthusiastic responses or contributions. If it did, then nurses would be organizing recreational programmes rather than therapeutic ones. It may be regarded, however, as a useful exercise to carry out in order to identify the poverty of their social skills and confirm the need for promoting them. One practical way of doing this is to ask patients specific questions about their personal hobbies and interests *before* they become involved in any organized group activity programmes. The statements made by patients during these interviews may be regarded as a 'baseline' measurement of their expressed interests. After a few weeks of regular participation in group activities, a similar set of interviews with the same patients can be repeated. Comparison between the two sets of interviews, before and after activities have been introduced, may produce some interesting results. An increase in the number and variety of statements relating to likes and dislikes may indicate a patient's favourable progress in expressing opinions on this particular subject.

If this idea is considered worthy of pursuing, then attempts should be made to structure these interviews as systematically as possible in order to obtain consistent and reliable data. It is important, for example, that all interviews be conducted privately and not in the hearing of other patients waiting to be interviewed. The necessity for this privacy is because many long-stay patients tend to be influenced by what they hear others say and frequently repeat what they immediately overhear. This may be regarded as an 'escape' behaviour. That is, it enables patients to give short relevant replies and escape from the more stressful situation of having to make a concentrated effort to think carefully before expressing their own personal views and opinions. In order to avoid this 'contamination' effect, in addition to the need for privacy in these interviews, the interviewer should be careful to avoid influencing the answers given by patients by suggesting to them the range of activities which are available. One way this influence may operate is by wording the questions in the form of a checklist of activities.

'Do you like playing darts?'—'Yes'.
'Do you like music?'—'Yes, I like music'.
'Do you like reading?'—'Yes'.

These types of question reduce the patient's need to think and restrict opportunities to give more personally relevant replies. It may also result in some patients saying 'Yes' more frequently than 'No', for some patients have learned from experience that to say 'Yes' to such questions reduces the time of their exposure to social contact, whereas a reply of 'No' to a question like 'Do you enjoy talking to people?' may invite a further question, 'Why don't you like talking to people?' which prolongs the interview and makes it more aversive.

The more 'open' type of question like 'What are your hobbies?', 'What games do you play?', are preferable because they allow greater scope for the patient to reply. These questions should also be standardized in the sense that identical questions should be asked of each patient at each set of interviews irrespective of the interval of time which may elapse between interviews. One way of doing this is to write out the questions and describe the conditions in which the interview should be conducted. In this way a 'standardized interview' can be produced.

The responsibility for planning and conducting group activity programmes for long-stay patients will depend a great deal on the nurses who usually look after them on the ward. These are the nurses who can best ensure continuity of treatment and care. The particular subjects in which staff are personally interested may form the foundation of a varied activity programme. Nurses who are enthusiastic about their special subjects are the obvious choice of person to organize them. As group leaders of these sessions, they are more likely to transmit their enthusiasm to patients and involve them in these activities than nurses who conduct them because they happen to be the only ones on duty. Consulting next week's duty sheet, therefore, must be considered an essential part of planning an activity programme. If an outdoor event has been planned to take place a few days ahead, it is always wise to plan also for an alternative indoor activity for the same period—unless all the staff have complete faith in the stability of the weather! Having to think of an alternative indoor activity on the spur of the moment may be a useful test of a nurse's initiative, but if it occurs too frequently it defeats the object of planning programmes.

The ward staff need to hold regular meetings to discuss the many aspects involved in planning these programmes, and the person in charge of the ward will, most likely, be the most suitable person to act as chairman and co-ordinator of this team project. The following paragraphs deal with some of the aspects to be reviewed when planning group activity programmes.

Duration

Taking into account the probability that many patients in the group will have problems related to concentration (i.e. the patient's span of continuous attention will be severely limited), the question arises of how long each activity should last. The rule of 'not too much and not too soon' provides a useful guideline to follow. Two 20 minutes sessions, with a 10–15 minute break in between, may be a suitable length of time to start with. If this period of time is found to be satisfactory, then it can gradually be extended to one which is regarded as ideal for a particular activity.

Frequency

After deciding how long an activity should last, the question arises of how many activities should be introduced in one week or even in one day. The same guidelines of moderation should apply. It is advisable to build up from a modest start and increase the number of activity sessions over time, rather than run the risk of subjecting patients to stress levels with which they are unable to cope. If we remember that emphasis in treatment should always be placed on what a patient can do, telling him what he has achieved and complimenting him on it, then it is more likely he will achieve the targets set if they are *gradually* upgraded. The problems of duration and frequency of activities need to be considered together rather than independently, for there must be a fairly calculated balance between them in order to achieve the best results. 'Feedback' on this subject will come from the behavioural responses of the patients.

Variety

A wide range of different types of subject and events will certainly make an activity programme more interesting. A variety of subjects concentrated into one week will impress the senior staff and visitors to the hospital, which may reinforce the ward nurses to maintain this pattern of activity programme. Unfortunately, it may have an adverse effect on some patients and be aversive. Though it may be true that a programme of stimulating events for regressed long-stay patients is just what the psychiatrist ordered, overstimulation for certain patients may prove to be antitherapeutic. One activity programme for the week contained a visit to a seaside resort, a trip to an agricultural show, a tour around the television studios, two sessions attending cricket matches, a visit to a speedway racing track, and a night out at a local club. For the next 3 weeks most patients walked around the ward in a daze. The impact of this concentrated stimulation introduced at too early a stage of the group activity programme resulted in many of them being out of touch with their immediate environment on the ward. Progressing treatment programmes, related to personal care of clothing and hygiene, deteriorated considerably, and a number of patients displayed some bizarre behaviours which had lain dormant for many years.

When returning to home and work after an enjoyable holiday, most of us respond in a similar, if less spectacular, manner to these patients. It does take a period of time to readjust to daily routine conditions, and the daily activity programmes should be modelled on the kind of balanced programme they are likely to continue after treatment ceases. Few of us are able continually to be on holiday nor would we desire to be. Variety may be the 'spice of life', but we can all appreciate it better when taken in small quantities spaced out over a period of time.

Patient involvement

Patient participation in the subject of the activity may be the major target for the group leader, but there are a number of subsidiary targets for the patient to achieve as he develops improved skills. These targets relate to helping the group leader to prepare for the activity, assisting during the activity and, eventually, taking over the activity for either part of the time or for the whole period. Patients rarely have the opportunity to practise behaviours related to organizing and planning events for others; the group leaders should be on the look-out for those who show some potential to do this and give them the opportunity to try. The ideal pattern of a group activity programme is that it should start with the nurses organizing and conducting it and end up by patients being responsible for it. After experiencing a range of activities over many weeks, patients will be more likely to take over and be responsible for part of the activity programme and help to plan as well as suggest future events.

Measuring and monitoring

If group leaders are to become therapists rather than masters of ceremonies, they need to know a great deal about their patients' behavioural problems before they can begin to conduct treatments in a group setting. Many of the patients' problems may have been recently identified and assessed before they started to attend group activities. If so, the group leader must seek out this valuable information to discover what the patient is like now, before group treatment begins. For the behavioural problems which have not been adequately assessed, the group setting may be an ideal place in which to measure them and obtain a 'baseline'. Most of the procedures, as well as the techniques previously described relating to individual programmes, also apply to treatments in a group setting.

Each session of a group activity is usually planned to last for a specific period of time. The classification of the activity under one of two categories will depend on the nature of the activity and the time available to complete it. There are two types of activity sessions—complete activity sessions and continuous activity sessions.

Complete activity sessions are those sessions where the subject of the activity can be completed within the time available in a single session.

Continuous activity sessions are those where the subject of the activity can *not* be finished in a single session but requires a number of similar periods, conducted over a greater interval of time, to complete it.

The reason for differentiating between these two kinds of activity is because it raises some important points in the management of activity programmes. For example, a member of the staff who is keen on taking 'art' sessions may, as a group leader, structure the event as a complete activity session. This can be done by giving the group a simple drawing exercise which can be carried out in one session by even the slowest member of the group. In these circumstances, any assessments required to measure the performance of different skills related to the subject of the activity, can be completed within this session. Monitoring the progress of an individual patient can be done by comparing the results obtained in each complete activity session with the previous ones. Using this method, a number of measurements related to each session can be plotted on a chart in sequence of their occurrence. The same group leader, conducting another 'art' session at a later stage in the programme, may feel the patients are now ready to tackle a more challenging project and decide to engage them in a slightly more ambitious exercise which, by the nature of the task, must extend over a number of 'art' sessions. The information required in these circumstances needs to be far more extensive in order to preserve the continuity between each session. There is a need to know how much progress was made in the exercise and the particular difficulties each patient had during the session. Their problems may be the focus of attention for remedial action at the next 'art' activity. To keep all this information concerning a number of patients 'in mind' for a week or more, before the next session takes place, would be unreasonable. Because the memory is notoriously unreliable in retaining a great deal of information over long periods of time, written records are valuable aids. When two or more therapists are working with the same group of patients, they must communicate and co-ordinate their practice in order to avoid confusing the patients and to ensure continuity of the programme.

GROUP DISCUSSION

Of all behaviours performed by man, 'talking' must be regarded as the most important behaviour which distinguishes him from other species. Though other animals may use sound to communicate with each other, they fail to match the complexities of human language in either form or content. Even the non-verbal language of signs, gestures and facial expressions of human beings are more diverse and subtle than those of other forms of animal life. Talking is a learned behaviour, the rudiments of which take place early in life and occur well before reaching school age. The main features of this learning process can be identified in the child's imitation of sounds made by its mother or father, the social and physical attention given to the child by its teacher–parents for imitating sounds, and the repeated pairing of particular sounds with material objects, which eventually leads to understanding of sounds as words with meaning. One important aspect of talking behaviour is that it is practised in a group environment, and the first experience of a group environment for a child is its home and its parents. Like many other behaviours, talking behaviour is maintained by its practice, and the expression 'what you don't use, you lose', seems to contain an element of truth. Many long-stay psychiatric patients have problems related to speech, and because the behaviour of talking is of major importance in the life of all human beings, treatment of talking difficulties should have priority. The most suitable environment for treating these problems is that provided in the activity of group discussion.

A particular activity sometimes has one main behaviour which is predominantly associated with its performance. This main behaviour can be described as the *primary behaviour* of the activity.

The obvious primary behaviour of a group discussion is 'talking'. All other behaviours related to this activity, such as listening, occasional head-nodding, eye contact with the speaker, and other non-verbal responses, may be regarded as *secondary behaviours*. Because there is such a close link between these behaviours, all talking problems, whether primary or secondary behaviours, can be treated within this single group activity at the same time.

The nature and severity of the problems may vary considerably between patients, and it is possible to have as many different problems as there are patients in the group. Some members of the group may speak very little, some may talk incessantly. Other patients may only reply to 'closed' questions which require a monosyllabic answer such as a 'Yes' or 'No'. Irrelevant talk, or various kinds of nonsense speech may dominate the conversation of other patients. The volume of sound issuing from a patient may be so low as to be inaudible to others more than a foot away. Repeating words or sentences may be the major problem of another patient.

A patient's problem or combination of problems must be identified and measured before a treatment is attempted. The nurse responsible for conducting a group activity must know the specific problems of each patient before beginning the group discussion and, as group leader and therapist, be familiar with the relevant techniques in order to obtain the maximum value from this treatment session. Some of the problems may belong to the group of behaviours classified as 'deficiencies' and need to be built up or increased in frequency, while behavioural 'handicaps', such as expressing bizarre ideas, require to be reduced and eventually extinguished. Patients with extremely severe problems, such as mutism, can not be treated effectively in a group situation. They require the concentrated and individual attention which can be given in a 'one-to-one' environment; that is, one therapist to one patient. Once a minimal level of speech has been established in this individual programme, these patients can then join a group discussion activity to generalize their talking behaviour to people other than the therapist.

Subjects for discussion

What do you say to a patient after you have said 'Hello'? Nurses, as well as visitors to the hospital, often have great difficulty in engaging long-stay patients in conversation. They find even greater difficulty in maintaining it for any length of time. Talking to patients who rarely reply, or if they do speak, say things which are irrelevant or incomprehensible, is not a rewarding experience. The consequence of such unproductive meetings is that they eventually cease to take place. The extinction of this social behaviour of visitors and nurses towards unresponsive patients, leads to that sinister situation often described as a 'vicious circle'.

1. The patient has a problem (does not talk; talks very little; talks 'oddly').

2. All forms of help to solve the problem require the presence of another person, or persons, who need to meet and talk to him frequently.

3. Because the patient has this problem, people avoid him.

4. Because people avoid him, he is deprived of the opportunity of help. Thus, his problem is perpetuated.

When an organized group of people get together to talk, they usually have a particular subject to talk about. This subject may be regarded as the purpose of their meeting.

Members of a football team may meet to talk about last Saturday's match and the reasons why they lost by six goals. From this inquest may develop a discussion on tactics for next week's encounter. Occasionally the talk may wander away from the main subject, but whenever it drifts too far, the manager of the team will usually channel it back. The purpose of this discussion is to improve the football skills of its members. Nurses may attend a management committee meeting to talk about hospital problems and find solutions. Though the items discussed may be varied, all topics are linked by the common theme of 'hospital problems'. It is the chairman of the committee who has the formal duty to ensure the boundaries of the subject are not exceeded. The purpose of this group discussion is to improve the efficiency of managing the hospital, which is the concern of all its members.

All members of similar groups have common interests and shared experiences, and it is these aspects which bring them periodically together to talk to each other for a particular purpose.

Many psychiatric patients are 'loners'. Despite the fact that they live in the same ward, eat at the same table, and sit next to each other in the lounge, they rarely communicate with each other. They are like 'ships that pass in the night'. Unlike recently admitted patients in psychiatric or general hospitals, they do not discuss their problems or ailments with each other. For long-stay patients those days have long since past. To gather a number of people into a single room for the purpose of talking may be regarded as the first step necessary to organize this activity, but it will not automatically transform them into a group, nor will group discussion inevitably take place. All patients need to participate regularly in the same programme of planned group activities, which should be as varied as possible, *before* a group discussion session is attempted. It is these other activities which provide the common interests and shared experiences so necessary to make talking behaviour more likely and provide subjects for discussion. When group discussion involves decision making, such as planning next week's activities, then it also has a well-defined purpose. Though talking problems may be generally considered to require priority in treatment of behavioural problems, this treatment should first be related to the daily events on the ward. Nurses should structure their interactions with patients in a way that provides frequent opportunities for them to talk and communicate. Group discussion sessions must be regarded as a more advanced form of treatment and their introduction into the activity programme should come at a later stage of treatment.

Structuring the environment

There are two ways in which we can structure an environment. One form applies to the way we deliberately change or arrange physical objects within a particular setting, and the other applies to the way we consciously use and adapt our personal approaches when talking to different people. The purpose of both forms of 'structuring the environment' is to provide a setting in which specific behaviours are made more likely to happen. The target behaviour for group discussion is 'appropriate talking', and all changes made in the area where this activity is to take place must be made with the idea of promoting this behaviour.

A suitable way to begin structuring the environment for group discussion sessions is to arrange the chairs in a circle. Though the concept of a circle has symbolic associations related to ideas of unity, harmony and eternity, due to the fact it has no beginning and no end, it is because of its practical application that a circular seating arrangement is chosen. All members of a group who sit in a circle can see each other quite clearly, are sitting in the most comfortable and convenient position to turn and talk with any other member of the group with the minimum of physical strain, and can become the leader of the group without formally changing the position of their seat. In order to promote the talking behaviour of a group of people, certain conditions must be present. People must be facing the speaker and the distance between speaker and listeners should be neither too near nor too far away. Occasional eye-contact must be exchanged between them, and there should be as little distraction as possible which might interrupt the continuity of the group discussion. Once these conditions have been achieved, it is the quality of the group leader's skills which will decide the development and progress of this group discussion as a treatment session.

Group leader's skills

The position of the group leader of an activity session is similar to that of a conductor of an orchestra. Just as some instruments need to be muted while others are required to play as loudly as possible, so garrulous patients need to be toned down and the timid socially withdrawn member of the group continually invited to talk more. Sufficient time must be given to each member of the group, and for this reason the maximum number should not exceed 12. When a group of patients have multiple speech problems requiring more intensive treatment, it may be necessary to reduce this maximum number to six or eight people in order to spend more time with each member.

Knowing the number of times a patient speaks during the group discussion, to whom he addresses his remarks, noting if he initiates the conversation or simply replies to a remark made by another person in the group, identifying his conversation as relevant or 'off the point', and being aware of the length of sentences he speaks may be some of the interesting information you, as a group leader, will require to measure a patient's progress in a group discussion activity. The group leader will, obviously, be unable to record this detailed information at the same time as he conducts the activity; he will require a colleague to assist him. This colleague should act as the assessor and sit in the background and never form part of the circle. If it is a person who is known to the patients and he frequently attends these activity sessions, his presence will become accepted and will be less likely to influence the behaviour of the group.

One way in which he can measure the social interactions of patients in the group, is in the form of a sociogram. The position of each person in the group is plotted on the assessment paper, including that of the group leader. Each time a member of the group makes a remark, a line is drawn from that person's plotted position to the position of the person he is addressing. To distinguish between which of two people initiated the remark, an arrow is placed on the end of the line in the direction of the person who is being addressed;

Example: 0   0
            Patient ◀━━━━━━━━━━ Patient
              (A)   (B)

In this example, patient (B) initiated a remark to patient (A). If patient (A) replies, then an arrow can be placed somewhere along the same line, but *not* placed at the end of it.

Example: 0   0
            Patient 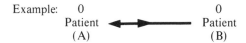 Patient
            (A)   (B)

Each line, complete with arrows, will indicate which people spoke, to whom they spoke, who initiated the conversation and if the person to whom they spoke replied. If the verbal interaction between two patients is repeated, lines parallel to the existing ones may be drawn which will indicate the number of interactions between those two particular people.

An overall picture of the discussion session can be drawn which will give the group leader an indication of the patterns of these interactions. When first starting group discussions, the group leader will have to perform a great deal of the work by speaking. The pattern of the sociograms will, most likely, prove it by showing that most of the remarks made during the sessions were made and initiated by the group leader. Conversations initiated by others will probably be found to have been directed mainly to the group leader. As the discussion sessions continue and the group leader encourages particular patients to talk more and his own contributions become less, the patterns of the sociograms will, hopefully, change. The patient who never stopped talking should now show a considerable reduction in lines and arrows. The patient who rarely spoke should now have an increased number of lines as well as a few arrows for initiating conversation. More people should be engaged in conversation and the direction of the lines and arrows should now be moving away from the position of the group leader and criss-crossing fairly equally over all parts of the circle. As the more capable patients are invited to take over the group discussion periods for an increasing amount of time, the nurse should be making preparations to fade out the role as group leader, intervening only when necessary to encourage and support members of the group.

During group sessions, the targets of all patients should be gradually up-graded. Reinforcements given to a patient who regularly replied to questions with a single word should next be required to give a two, three- or four-word reply before receiving the same reinforcer. At a later stage in the programme the same patient may be judged to be capable of initiating speech and will only receive his reinforcer when he does so. Judgements regarding what a patient is capable of doing and decisions relating to changes in his programme and when those changes should be made, are dependent on the experience of the group leader. What the group leader should not be afraid of doing is to go back a stage in a patient's programme if the patient can not meet the demands made by the upgrading.

We all have a potential and we also have a limit. In order to find out what our potential or limit is, we have to put it to the test. We must remember that our job in a group discussion activity is not to make the patients who form the group great orators or even gregarious people. It is to help them reach the limits of their potential in the behaviour of speech as a method of expression and communication. The aim of some discussion groups is to invite and encourage its members to focus their attention on their own behavioural problems as well as comment and give their views of the behaviour of other members of the group. Such groups consist of people who are sufficiently articulate to express opinions and in time, as they become better acquainted, their conversation becomes more uninhibited and they are less reluctant to talk about their problems. The aim of discussion groups for long-stay patients may very well be to reduce the frequency of uninhibited conversations expressed by some of its members, to divert attention from their problems associated with bizarre ideas and obsessional behaviours, and to concentrate attention on the 'reality' aspect of life. It is more important for long-stay patients to be aware of what is happening in their immediate external environment and to extend their boundaries of reality to the world outside the hospital. The repeated practice of directing attention from self to external realities may establish behaviours which are incompatible with their behavioural deficiencies and handicaps.

A WALKING ACTIVITY

With the exception of people who have been confined indoors for a considerable time, there is very little that is exciting about going for a walk. That is, unless there is a special motive for doing so. When the reason is to explore the countryside, enjoy the views, to bird watch, or to visit the local pub, it gives added purpose and joy to the journey. A walk in the hospital grounds for many patients in the past was a privilege and a favourite item on the activity programme of long ago. Perhaps the main disadvantage from the patient's point of view was the fact it could only take place in the company of many other patients and always under the eagle eye of the nurse–attendant escort. The choice of wandering at will, or deciding the route, or even pausing to examine a particularly interesting object, was the nurse's privilege, not the patients'. The main aim of the activity was to get the patients off the ward and out into the fresh air for a fixed amount of time. The purpose of the walking activity was to promote their physical health.

Any nurse who answered the question: 'What are the advantages of a walk in the hospital grounds for mental patients?' with: 'This exercise is beneficial to patients because it gives tone to their muscles, expands their lungs, improves their respiratory and circulatory systems, and thereby stimulates their appetite. If sufficient energy has been expended during the exercise, then aggressive tendencies may be reduced and night sedations are less likely to be required.'—This nurse was most likely to pass the hospital examination. The fact that all these physical benefits would be present if the walk also had a purpose other than the exercise itself was of less concern in those days. The silence of the patients, as they walked in a 'crocodile' line with one nurse at the front and one at the back of the line, was considered to be part of their mental illness. As they never appeared to take an interest in anything around them as they walked, the only value of the walk seemed to be the exercise.

Commenting on this piece of history, a third-year student nurse said, 'It's still true. I've recently seen patients walking together with heads down and eyes fixed on the ground. They walk in the same group but don't appear to belong to it. They may look at things but they don't seem to take much notice of them and they rarely speak to each other. I don't think there is much more value for them in a walk than the benefits of the exercise.' The student was invited by the charge nurse to accompany him on a short walk in the hospital grounds with a number of long-stay patients, and asked to observe the patients carefully.

On returning to the ward, the student was asked for his impressions and observations of the walk activity. 'It merely confirmed the things I said previously', he replied. 'All the patients appeared solitary, engaged in their own thoughts, and none of them spoke to each other. They didn't appear to take much interest in their environment and, beyond the benefit of the physical exercise, the outside event didn't provide them with much stimulation.'

After the staff and patients had drunk their cups of tea, they were all asked by the charge nurse to sit down and start a group discussion. The first topic for discussion was the walk. The first patient to speak mentioned that a banner had been put up in the hospital grounds to advertise the annual hospital fête, which was due to take place in a week's time. The next patient said he also saw it, and repeated the exact words he had seen printed on the banner. As the banner had been facing the public highway, and as our route had taken us behind the banner, the letters on the sign could only be seen in reverse, like 'mirror' writing. One patient mentioned he noticed the large grass roller on the sports field was a bit rusty, another reported he saw a young woman being helped into an ambulance by an ambulance driver near the general hospital. Further observations by different patients were meeting a student nurse who had worked on the ward 6 months previously, and repeating the verbal exchanges between that student and the charge nurse. There were many other pieces of information directly related to the walk which patients spoke about. Because the charge nurse and the student nurse had been present at this event, they were able to confirm the patients' statements of what they had seen and heard as true. The student admitted that his interpretation of the patients' behaviour, though based upon his own observations, had been proved to be wrong.

There is a great deal we need to know about our patients, particularly the therapeutic value of engaging them in specific activities. If we intend to use activities as stimuli to arouse their interest and curiosity, it is important we find out if we have succeeded. It would be helpful to know, not only how many events or incidents attracted their attention (the frequency of their responses to stimuli), but also to know which parts of an activity attracted their interest most (the strength of specific stimuli). In this activity of 'a walk in the hospital grounds', we found our observations of the patients' behaviour useful but incomplete. We also became aware that to use our observations alone to interpret their behaviour could lead to wrong conclusions. More information was obviously required to supplement our observations before we could assess its value as a stimulating event. This additional evidence was found in our 'follow-up' activity of a group discussion.

It appears there are at least three sources from which information can be obtained: (1) what patients say, (2) what patients do, and (3) what the therapist observes.

When all these sources of information correlate, the evidence may be considered reliable.

DRAMA ACTIVITY

> All the world's a stage,
> And all the men and women merely players;
> They have their exits and their entrances;
> And one man in his time plays many parts . . . .

Long-stay patients in hospital do not play many parts. Their role is usually confined to that of 'patient'; the scene in which they play it is usually a 'hospital' setting. Even when they leave the hospital and the scene is changed to 'a town centre', or 'inside a store', they still continue to act their part of 'patient', and can often be identified by members of the public in this particular role.

The use of drama, or play-acting sessions, can be useful in stimulating real-life scenes and situations in which patients can practise a variety of roles which most of us play every day of our lives. After patients have acquired the social skills necessary in these different situations, they need to transfer their performance from the rehearsal area of the simulated scene to the 'real-life' stage. The more accomplished the performance, the more likely they are to be accepted as other members of the community and treated as such. We may not be conscious of the roles we play during our daily routine, but when we direct our attention to them, they appear in very sharp focus. In the scene, 'Home', we may play the part of a parent, and depending upon which gender of the species we are, we may also play the part of a son or daughter, wife or husband, elder or younger brother or sister, the lodger, a guest, or the host. When the milkman knocks on the door, we become customers, and if we are in control of the household finances, we act our parts as chancellors of the exchequer. The 'Street' scene may provide us with an opportunity to change our role to a pedestrian, a motorist, or passenger on a bus or train. The purchase of a daily newspaper will help us to keep in touch with local and national events so we are able to contribute to a discussion with other people, or at least to understand what they are talking about. Though the newspaper cannot be regarded as the script from which we learn our lines, it can be looked upon as the background material we require to interact with other people, whether it be as speaker or listener. The scene, 'At work', provides us with another setting in which our variety of roles is extended. As employees in a hospital environment, we may act as figures of authority one moment, giving instructions to other employees, and a few minutes later we may be taking and carrying out instructions from another employee with a different status and function. We may have a part as a teacher of nurses in the morning, and that of a student learning from other nurses in the afternoon. Dining in the hospital canteen with our colleagues, we become customers again, and as diners we become entitled to express our opinions concerning the food to the chef or catering officer.

As people in our home, on the public highway, or at work, there is no doubt we play many parts in the space of one day. Though we may choose to play our different roles in a set way as we interact with other people in our private life, in our role as 'nurse' to the person known as 'the patient' we must be aware of the danger of becoming too fixed and stereotyped. We need to be particularly flexible enough to act out many parts with our patients. Even with a single patient, our role must change appropriately as the occasion arises. If we intend to be involved in his rehabilitation, then we must be prepared to take on the roles of teacher, adviser and counsellor, and as a friend, at different times. One way which can help us to adapt ourselves to these different aspects of our role as 'nurse' is to use the settings provided by the various activities, and to use them in the most imaginative and productive way possible. Drama group sessions can substitute for real-life scenes and cater for situations not covered by the daily routine of the ward or any of the other group activities. One of the functions of drama group sessions is to help the patient to increase the number of roles he can play in life, and to help him to perform those roles with as great a skill as possible.

An equally important function of drama group activities is to concentrate on the specific behavioural problems of individual patients which may be the obstacles to learning or practising skills.

Many talking behaviours can, of course, be treated within a group discussion, but as it is often said, 'We talk not only with our voices, but also our bodies'. The way we move, the gestures we make, and the facial expressions we use, represent a body language which, if appropriately synchronized with our voice, can emphasize and illustrate the content of our conversation more vividly. The main advantage which drama sessions have over discussion groups is that people can move about and extend their skills in social interactions. A group discussion is a sitting activity and because talking behaviours occur in situations other than sitting positions, drama sessions can be regarded as ideal settings in which the behaviour of talking can be further developed.

It is possible to concentrate on body language as a specific subject on its own. For people who have particular difficulties in posture and movement, it is an aspect of drama which can be extremely useful to them. A whole branch of the theatre is devoted to this art form in the subject of Mime and Dance. A useful exercise for patients who always deliver their speech in dull monotones (flatness of affect), or giggle at serious situations and frown at amusing ones (incongruity of affect), is to play parts in a specially written sketch containing a variety of situations which are designed to evoke specific emotional responses. The use of this mini-play allows the group leader to concentrate attention on these problems under controlled conditions. For the hyperactive patient, whose problem is continual 'pacing', a role as a wax model in a Tussaud's exhibition may be appropriate. In succeeding sketches he can be allowed to play parts which extend his range of movement. For the patient who always whispers, a part as a court-usher or town-crier may help to raise the level of his voice. Arranging for him to engage in a conversation with another patient with a great distance between them may increase the volume.

It is obvious that there cannot be a single method or procedure which will suit all patients. We cannot design treatments for behavioural problems; we can only design treatments for *people* who happen to have specific behavioural problems. This means that nurse–therapists may need to experiment with a wide range of ideas before they can hit upon the most appropriate method or technique for a particular patient. There are, however, a number of general rules which are worth keeping in mind. Patients playing roles which are incompatible with their behavioural problems, is a good one to follow. The socially withdrawn and compliant patient should play parts of authority in which he can practise being assertive. The aggressive type of patient, the quiet and more humble roles. Those who fear the venture may be so successful that the timid person may change into an aggressive personality and the dominating patient into a completely submissive one may rest assured. There is no report of this ever happening with psychiatric patients participating in a drama group session. The best result the group leader can expect is their problem behaviours will be gradually modified by the constant practice of the opposite type of behaviour, and that is the result required. One important point to remember is not to gradually build up or tone down these roles, but to start them off playing extreme parts from the very beginning. This is part of the method called 'overlearning'—a method whereby there is a tendency for the patient to go past his appropriate target, but with the passage of time he settles down to a level which is generally regarded as normal behaviour. Another general rule is to keep the whole group active all of the time. While the group leader may be occupied for a time concentrating on the performance of two or three patients, the attention of the other members of the group may wander. If there is nothing specific for them to do, it is as well to invite them to become an active audience by asking them to take special notice of the performers 'on stage' and to give their comments at frequent intervals. Another general rule which should be followed is that no unexpected visitors should be allowed to enter the rehearsal area and interrupt the continuity of a drama workshop session. If visitors do enter, it should be by previous invitation in consultation with the other members of the group, and they should preferably come to the activity as participators rather than onlookers.

THE PLAY

Many organizers of drama sessions may prefer the more conventional approach to this activity by wanting to produce a published play. As a project to stage eventually before an audience it may be regarded as an exceptionally ambitious plan for patients with problems of posture, movement, and a variety of speech disabilities. For patients without any gross disabilities, it may be an excellent idea if certain points are kept in mind. It would, for example, be wise to start with a one-act rather than a three-act play; a play with a running time of 30 minutes as opposed to one that lasts an hour and a half will stand a better chance of achieving a public performance. The behaviours of learning lines, remembering cues to enter or speak, painting the set, making the 'props', making and wearing the costumes on dress rehearsal night, produce the same excitement and require the same skills as a full-length play—but make the venture more feasible.

The choice of the play is critical from two points of view, that of the patients and that of the therapist. Whether it be tragedy or comedy, the value of the play lies in its content. The greater the patients' interest and understanding of the play, linked with the relevance of it to their personal lives, the greater its therapeutic value. A play which requires a patient who repeatedly says 'off-stage', 'I own this hospital, I'm the richest man in the world', to act the part of the King of Siam, cannot be regarded as helpful to the patient from a treatment point of view. Likewise, a patient who has a problem related to persecutory ideas should not play a part like Shylock, in *The Merchant of Venice*. If we cannot extinguish or reduce such behaviours, we should be careful not to strengthen or increase them. Awareness of one's own behaviour and its possible consequences is an important attribute of a behavioural therapist's skill. Another important point to remember is that not all patients who have problems related to posture or movement, such as rigidity or excessive slowness or quickness in walking, have these signs because of environmental or psychopathological causes. They may well be due to the 'side-effects' of drugs, or even the beginning of a physical illness. It is for this reason that nurse–therapists should always consult the ward doctor and 'screen' such a patient before proceeding with a behavioural treatment.

A further extension of the idea of putting on a play for presentation to an audience was that undertaken by a group of long-stay patients in co-operation with their group leader. They all decided not only to produce a play, but also to write it themselves. The play was based on one of their weekly activities—a visit to the local town where they did their personal shopping and stopped at a coffee bar for light refreshment. One of the places they liked to visit was the outdoor market, and this was one of the scenes they decided as a setting for the opening of their play. The plot was based on the character of a stallholder selling leather suitcases and hand-bags who, while his back was turned, was robbed of a brief-case by a 'shifty' character who had been hanging about the market stall. The discovery of the theft by the tradesman, the confrontation with the alleged thief, the calling of a policeman, and the involvement of a witness, resulted in scene two, 'A magistrate's court'. This scene naturally introduced several other characters into the play in the form of the court officials. The background material for the market scene was well known to the cast, that of the court was unfamiliar. It was decided, therefore, to arrange a visit to the local court for a few of the patients, and so the event became an activity on the weekly programme.

The situations within this play, if simple in form, were certainly dramatic in content, and the words needed to express these characters' feelings were plain to the point of bluntness. The dialogue was based on the 'free-expression' of the patients as they acted out their respective roles. That is, they were given the outline of a particular situation by the group leader and, as they kept the characters they were playing in mind, they said to each other what they felt at the time. As they delivered their 'lines' during these encounters, their words and sentences were written down by a member of the staff and used as a basic pattern to structure the dialogue of the play. After the group had discussed the dialogue and made their alterations and amendments, it was typed and duplicated in manuscript form. As soon as the members had received their copies of the play, the rehearsals began.

Besides concentrating on the way the patients expressed their lines, the group leader also involved them in discussion. He would stop the play at particular points and ask the cast, 'Is this the way you would behave if you were wrongly accused of stealing?' To a reply of 'No' he would say, 'Then how would you act and what would you say and do?' Eventually someone would volunteer to replace the actor cast in the part, who would sit in the audience as his understudy gave his version of the character. If his understudy's interpretation was convincing, the player would repeat the scene in an attempt to model himself on the performance recently given.

'Do you think the magistrate is playing his part too much like an American judge in a film of a murder trial?' 'Is the defence laywer presenting a good case for the accused, or do you think it could be better?' were some of the interjections made by the group leader to stimulate patients' thinking in the hope of rational and logical responses. Tape recordings were made of many of the rehearsals and played back to them immediately after the performance. This gave the patients an opportunity to talk about many aspects of their vocal talents which were not always complimentary. This novelty form of 'feedback' for the patients quite noticeably improved their subsequent performances. 'If only we had a video-recorder', mused the director of the play, 'we could also show the patients how they moved as well'!

Perhaps one day video-recorders for treatment purposes will become as standard equipment for nurse–therapists in psychiatric hospitals as the drug cupboard fitted in every ward today. Meanwhile, the show must go on. The patients gave two performances before fellow patients in adjoining wards, and achievement was reflected in their faces.

OTHER GROUP ACTIVITIES

There are a considerable number of other interesting subjects which can be utilized as group activities to the advantage of the patient's treatment. These include:

Creative activities such as drawing, painting, model making, thread sculpture, and collages, pottery, woodwork and jewellery making.

Educational programmes to teach patients domestic skills such as washing, ironing and sewing, as well as household tasks like mending a fuse and how to wire an electric plug. Money and its related subjects— budgeting and saving—may be some of the relevant topics that need to be covered for a particular group of patients.

Indoor/outdoor games and sports can provide a host of ideas to stimulate patients and give them opportunities to plan and organize many of these events themselves. To these subjects can be added music, quiz sessions, dances and out-of-hospital trips.

All of these subjects are worthy of discussion in their own right. Within the space of a single chapter, however, it is impossible to investigate their particular qualities in any great depth, or to the level they deserve. Some general comments applying to all activities, and a few opinions on particular subjects, may be helpful to those who have little experience of activities as more than pastimes.

Music

There are specialists in this subject who insist that in order to use music as a therapy one must possess qualifications in music and be a qualified teacher as well. If the purpose is to teach a patient to play a musical instrument, to read music, or to gain a technical appreciation of music, then most people would support this claim. When a patient is discovered to have played a musical instrument as a hobby, or relied on it for his living, the value of a music therapist in treating this patient is beyond dispute. As well as the common interest between the patient and the therapist, and the opportunity provided by this meeting for the patient to renew his interest and improve his skill, there is always hope that it may lead to rehabilitation in the community.

When the services of a full-time music therapist are not available, and when most patients are interested in music, but at a less intensive level, the activity can still be a useful subject for group sessions, and can be structured in many different ways. There is a body of opinion which supports the idea of giving the patients what they ask for, or giving them the types of music they say they like. This is done in the sincerely held belief that it is of greater therapeutic value to the patient, and as a general rule this appears to be so.

There was, however, one occasion when there was an exception to this rule. A young nurse volunteered to take over a music session, but had been unable to obtain the records previously ordered from the public library. In order not to disappoint the patients, she brought to the group activity some of her own 'pop' records and apologized for playing them because, as she said, 'That's all I've got'. As the average age of the patients in the group was 46 years, she did not expect them to be received with the same enthusiasm as herself—and she was right!

Whereas previous sessions had induced increasing lethargy and, as a consequence, less discussion, when the 'pop' records were played this group became suddenly alert. Instead of being lulled by melodious Viennese waltzes they were shocked into paying attention, and in the group discussion periods between records there was no need for the group leader to encourage them to speak. 'Too loud!', 'Too harsh!', 'A load of rubbish!' were the kind of remarks passed. No, it is not always beneficial to take along music that we think the group will like. Sometimes it is more therapeutic to use music which is 'unusual' to them.

Playing the type of music which is familiar to patients often triggers off memories which, in turn, can provide subjects for the talking periods in between the records played. If 'talking' is one of the behaviours the group leader wishes to encourage, then restricted use of long-play records is advisable. Here is an example where *pre-planning* of an activity (in terms of deciding the number of musical items, the time allowed for playing, and the kinds of behavioural responses the therapist desires to increase) can be critical in producing favourable results.

Art

In a similar way to music, the subject of art as a therapy has its supporters as well as its qualified practitioners. There is an obvious advantage in using this medium for patients who have difficulties in verbal communication. The danger lies in interpreting some of their work and using it to assist in the diagnosis of mental illness. A visitor interpreted one particular painting as 'typically schizophrenic'. The sheet of paper upon which brilliant colours had been painted and arranged in fascinating patterns was nothing more than a staff nurse's random testing of some paints which had arrived from the hospital stores that morning. A painting of a man dressed in black standing against a very dark blue background was identified as the work of an 'extremely depressed' patient. The group leader who was in charge of the session when this particular painting was done would have been able to give the reason for the colours used, but maintained a polite silence. They happened to have been the only colours which were available at the time!

The teaching of techniques and improving the skills of patients is certainly the province of the expert, but for long-stay patients who have some interest but little talent, the act of doing it may be sufficient reward. The therapist can still measure the result of their pleasure which may provide him with additional information. The amount of attention patients pay to their immediate environment may be an aspect of behaviour which the therapist would like to assess. The use of an art activity may be a very useful way of discovering this information. A nurse conducting an art session asked the group members to draw a picture of the dining room, with the tables set for dinner. When their drawings had been completed, the nurse collected and reviewed them later. By counting the numbers of relevant items drawn by each patient in his picture, the nurse obtained some idea of the 'attention to environment' behaviour of every patient. True, some of the squiggles and lines were difficult to decipher, but the problem was always solved by asking the patient.

It is always worth while to practise analysing all activities in terms of their primary and secondary behaviours. One can then match these main behaviours necessary to practise the activities with the patient's problem behaviour. By using this approach, the group leader will be able to choose the activities which suit the patients best and provide the most ideal settings for treatment.

Gardening

A gardening activity, such as flower and vegetable cultivation, may seem an attractive proposition. Yet one must consider a number of factors in choosing a gardening activity before one can take full advantage of its possibilities in terms of treatment and rehabilitation.

For one or two patients who seem to be extremely interested in the subject, it may lead to attending evening leisure classes held in this subject in the local town. If they regularly attend these sessions and talk enthusiastically about them when they return to the ward, it could lead to a further stage in rehabilitation. If they have been assessed as having potential to live in the community, one can think in terms of possible employment in this line. A job associated with market gardening, work with the Parks department of the local authority, or as a self-employed freelance gardener, may all be future possibilities for patients who have great interest in this subject.

If the patient's chance of discharge is low, then the value of the activity as a treatment is considerably reduced. Gardening cannot be described as an ideal group activity, but for an individual patient who has been treated in a group environment, it may open up an avenue to discharge from hospital. Though gardening is a creative activity, its results and its rewards are far from immediate. The long time-delay between behaviour and its consequences is a disadvantage from a treatment point of view. Should the staff decide to feature 'gardening' as a regular group activity, then it must be remembered that it is also a 'continuous' activity which requires constant monitoring by an enthusiastic group leader. If the patients concerned have not yet developed sufficient initiative to look after their plots of land before the group leader goes on his 2 weeks' vacation, he may return to find his 'land of plenty' reduced to a 'barren waste'.

THE FINAL TARGET

'What do patients do when they no longer have nurse-organized activities?' The ideal answer should be, 'They organize the activities themselves'. In order to achieve this ultimate target, group leaders should always keep in mind the need gradually to increase the part played by patients in all activities, as they gradually decrease their own. An increasing number of sessions entitled 'Own choice', should appear each week in the group activity programme. The purpose of these 'Own choice' activities is to give patients an opportunity to organize their own leisure periods, and to enable group leaders to observe if behaviours learned during activity sessions generalize to these periods.

'Own choice' periods may be considered as the areas in which patients are able to demonstrate their progress in terms of functioning constructively on their own initiative. Whether the patients engage in recreational events with others, or indulge alone in a personal hobby, perform activities associated with self-care, write letters, or visit relatives is of little importance. What may be of greater significance if they have never previously exhibited these behaviours without direction and supervision from others, is that this may be an indication that they have taken their first step on the path to rehabilitation.

BIBLIOGRAPHY AND FURTHER READING LIST

Argyle M. (1970) *The Psychology of Interpersonal Behaviour.* Ch 2 and 6. Harmondsworth, Penguin.

Arieti S. (1979) *Understanding and helping the Schizophrenic.* Harmondsworth, Pelican Books.

Ayllon T. and Azrin M. (1968) *The Token Economy.* New York, Appleton-Century Crofts.

Barton R. (1976) *Institutional Neurosis.* Bristol, John Wright.

Beech H. R. (1969) *Changing Man's Behaviour.* Ch 8. Harmondsworth, Penguin.

Clark D. H. (1974) *Social Therapy in Psychiatry.* Ch 3 and 4. Harmondsworth, Penguin.

Cohen S. and Taylor L. (1972) *Psychological Survival.* Ch 2, 3, and 4. Harmondsworth, Penguin.

Crowcroft A. (1975) *The Psychotic.* Harmondsworth, Penguin.

Eisler R. M., Hersen M. and Miller P. M. (1973) Effects of modelling on components of assertive behaviour. *J. Behav. Ther. Exp. Psychiatry.* 4, 1–6.

Goffman E. (1970) *Asylums.* Ch 1. Harmondsworth, Penguin.

Jones M. (1968) *Beyond the Therapeutic Community.* New Haven, Conn. Yale U.P.

Lebow M. D. (1976) Applications of behaviour modification in nursing practice. In: Hersen M., Eisler R. M. and Miller P. M. (ed.) *Progress in Behaviour Modification,* Vol. 2. London, Academic Press.

Matson J. L. (1980) Behaviour modification procedures for training chronically institutionalized schizophrenics. In: Herson M., Eisler R. M. and Miller P. M. (ed.) *Progress in Behaviour Modification,* Vol. 9. London, Academic Press.

Morgan I. R. and Cheadle J. (1981) *Psychiatric Rehabilitation.* National Schizophrenic Fellowship, Surrey.

Priestley M. (1975) *Music Therapy in Action.* London, Constable.

Schaefer H. H. and Martin P. L. (1975) *Behavioural Therapy.* New York, McGraw-Hill.

Watts F. N. and Bennett D. H. (1983) *Theory and Practice of Psychiatric Rehabilitation.* New York, Wiley.

Wethered G. (1973) *Drama and Movement in Therapy.* London, McDonald & Evans.

Wing J. K. and Brown C. W. (1970) *Institutionalism and Schizophrenia.* Ch 1. London, Cambridge University Press.

Index